PRANIC LIVING AND HEALING

Prana has many levels of meaning from the breath to
the energy of consciousness itself. It is not only
the basic life-force, it is the master form of
all energy working on the level of mind, life
and body. Indeed the entireuniverse is
a manifestation of Prana, which
is the original creative power.
This book presents certain interesting reports and more
fascinating material on the subject of pranic
nourishment. It gives, side-by-side, all sides
of the picture to enable you to decide
for yourselves on the concerned issues.
However, there is much more to prana than just
nourishment. It has immense potential, which is
alsodiscussed in detail here. The book
provokes you to have your own
experiences with prana!

PRANIC LIVING
and
HEALING

Luis S. R. Vas

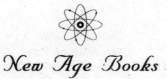

New Age Books

ISBN: 81-7822-161-6

First Edition: Delhi, 2003

Disclaimer
The readers are warned not to attempt any such pranic nourishment, as
mentioned in the book, except with the approval and under the
supervision of a qualified medical practitioner in view of the fatalities
that have been reported, through misjudgement or for any other reason.

Published by
NEW AGE BOOKS
A-44 Naraina Phase I
New Delhi-110 028 (INDIA)
Email: nab@vsnl.in
Website: www.newagebooksindia.com

Printed in India
at Shri Jainendra Press
A-45 Naraina Phase-I, New Delhi-110 028

Introduction

On April 14, 2002, I read the following report by Aruna Raghuram in *The Asian Age* which I reproduce below:

Diyas, incense and strewn rose petals. Enough to give that air of mysticism to the proceedings. The occasion: a seminar in Ahmedabad on "Living on Light". Puzzled? The seminar is addressed by an Australian woman Jasmuheen, who has gone without food for seven years!

For her eating a 'light' meal does not mean what it means to the rest of us – eating less, it means not eating at all. She has instead managed to tap the divine light within her. Still puzzled? Don't blame you. It sounds bizarre till you know a little more about it.

The practice she follows is called pranic nourishment and Jasmuheen says in the coming decades it may be the answer to global hunger and malnutrition. The technique developed by her combines ancient knowledge and spiritual wisdom with futuristic "biofield" science.

Anybody can live on light provided they follow an eight point plan to change their lifestyle. The eight points are–meditation, prayer, programming of the mind, vegetarian diet, exercise, time spent in silence, service to others and chanting. Following such a lifestyle tunes the "biofield" (energy vibrations created by the physical, mental and emotional patterns) of a person. "When a person's biofield is well tuned, he or she can access DOW (Divine One Within) power which will love, guide and heal the person and nourish the cells," she says.

Jasmuheen lives on water with a little lemon juice in it and an occasional cup of tea. Perhaps, once a week she may take some potato or cauliflower as a salad. On Christmas day, she indulges herself with a bowl of soup. That's it. She does not depend of food for nourishment.

It took Jasmuheen 20 years (she is now 45 years old) to prepare her body to live without food. "But now I've found the formula. It would take a person six months now to do it," she says. A person living on light can occasionally have something he loves like chocolates or ice-cream.

A group of Indians who are going to live on light will be tested on August 2003 by an Ahmedabad-based doctor, Dr. Sudhir Shah and his team. Dr. Sudhir Shah has been studying the case of 65-year-old Hira Ratan Manek of Ahmedabad who has survived on just solar energy for 411 days.

A new branch of science called neurotheology is studying how living on light affects the pituitary and pineal glands, says Jasmuheen.

"A pranically nourished person does not fall ill, has more energy, needs to sleep less and is able to maintain a stable weight," says Jasmuheen. To her knowledge there are 10,000 people the world over living on light. Many people keep it quiet because others may think they are crazy. The oldest person living on light is a 96-year-old woman.

Jasmuheen wants to give up water as well. However, a hectic travelling schedule makes it difficult. "Because of interacting with so many people and exposure to pollution, if I give up even water I would lose weight and become weak." To allay the fears of her family she gets a complete health check up every year.

Saranya Zaveri from Chennai has been living on light for the past year. She describes her 21-day initiation (which is not compulsory) into the practice. "The first seven days were the toughest as I had to go without even water. During that time I maintained silence and had several visions and I felt I was living in a different world. The last few days I was in tears and begged for a sip of water. My husband gave me support. 'You can do it,' he said. The next 14 days I could have water with a little juice in it. Before this initiation, I had prepared my body by going on a diet of salads and soups."

Actually, she explains, before living on light a person has to prepare his or her body by giving up different types of fruits in stages. In the first stage red meat, in the second all meat and dairy products and in the third cooked food, is given up. In the fourth stage only liquids are consumed. The fifth stage is that of living on light. Jasmuheen has also held seminars in Mumbai, Delhi, Chennai and Pondicherry.

I was intrigued by this story and decided to investigate the matter. I discovered that research had been done not only on prana but also on BIGU, a form of spontaneous fasting that some practitioners of Qi gong, a Chinese spiritual technique, undergo.

I also learnt that some people undergoing the 21-day initiation of living on light had died of dehydration. Jasmuheen however claims that they willfully and carelessly broke some of the rules of the initiation and suffered in consequence.

I read a report that Jasmuheen had been challenged by a TV programme in Australia to stay without food under their supervision but had 'failed' the test, according to the report's headline. But the report itself stated that the producers of the programme themselves had terminated the test because, although Jasmuheen claimed that she was feeling well, medical tests showed her dehydrating progressively and they would be held culpable in case anything untoward happened to her.

I also discovered a report on Hira Ratan Manek's 411 days of fast, certified by the doctors who had supervised his fast.

In this book, I present all this and more fascinating material on this subject of pranic nourishment, giving all sides of the picture to enable readers to decide for themselves on the concerned issues. I should however warn the readers not to attempt any such pranic nourishment except with the approval and under the supervision of a qualified medical practitioner in view of the fatalities that have been reported, through misjudgement or for any other reason.

But there is much more to prana than just nourishment. It has immense healing potential, which is also discussed in detail in this book. I look forward to hearing from readers on their experiences with prana.

LUIS S.R. VAS
vasluis@hotmail.com

Contents

CHAPTER 1

Hira Ratan Manek's 411-day Fasting Saga

The Times of India, dated December 30, 2000, carried a report titled **"Engineer uses sun to claim victory over hunger."** It is reproduced below:

AHMEDABAD: Can the human body turn into a photovoltaic cell and convert the rays of the sun into energy? Sixty-four-year-old retired mechanical engineer Hira Ratan Manek claims it can. For the past 364 days, he claims he has not swallowed a single morsel of solid, living only on some boiled water and the star closest from the earth.

"We humans live primarily on secondary solar energy as the plants which we consume depend heavily on the sun to grow," Manek, a Kutchi living in Coimbatore, says. "All you need to do is learn to absorb from the primary source of solar energy."

To ensure that Manek's story does not sound like a fairy tale, there are an array of doctors from the Health Care International Multitherapy Institute and the Jain Doctors Association who have been monitoring his health from two days before the fast started, which will last up to February 15 to complete 411 days.

The method of becoming a solar cooker is quite simple. According to Manek, you start by looking straight into the rising morning sun for only a few seconds.

Slowly you increase the time to minutes reaching up

to 30 to 35 minutes. "If you do it gradually, your eyes will not be damaged and help in charging your brain with solar energy."

Manek adds that once you go above 15 minutes, your desire for food slowly diminishes. "It is victory over hunger, not its suppression." At 30 to 35 minutes, the human brain starts developing the capacity to store solar energy.

"All you need to do is take a walk barefoot for about 40 to 45 minutes in the sun everyday to recharge the energy." Claims Manek, "Only through this process can man achieve complete freedom or Moksha. You rid yourself from physical and psychological ailments. Psychosomatic ailments out of stress become a distant dream.

But more importantly you develop a corona of energy around you. As this energy field becomes stronger, diseases don't harm you. Even your worst enemy will become harmless."

Eminent neuro-physician Sudhir Shah, who has been monitoring Manek's health with a team of doctors, says, "What we have is not 100 per cent science, but hypothesis. However, we believe that this is a chronic case of adaptation syndrome where the body reduces its demand for energy after 16 to 30 days of fasting. This is done by downing the regulation of receptors."

Shah does not rule out the possibility that the temporal lobe in the human brain, which is believed to control parapsychic activity like the sixth sense, may have been activated due to this process. All other parts of the brain including the hypothalamus, the pituitary glands and the medulla oblongata have shown no signs of changing.

For Manek, a Shwetambar Jain, the fast has both religious and scientific connotations. "All this search for a microchip to insert in the human brain to store loads of information and increase memory is ridiculous," he says. "We don't even use 10 per cent of it. But once charged, its capacity is increased manifold. In fact, enlightenment in spiritual terms is nothing but 100 per cent use of the brain!"

Hira Ratan Manek, a 63-year-old mechanical engineer and a Gujarati businessman, who has done fasting for 211 days during 19th June, 1995 to 15th January, 1996, has started yet another fast for 411 days from 1st January, 2000.

Hira Ratan Manek is following the Jain way of fasting and he takes only water after sunrise and before sunset from 1st January 2000. He became famous during 1996 when he started a fast for 211 days with only water. The fast which he started aiming at the prosperity of the world ended, in the Jain temple situated in Gujarat.

The medical team is led by Health Care International Multitherapy Institute and Jain Doctors Federation jointly. It is fully supported by Jain Yuvak Mahasangh President Dr. Jitubhai Shah.

"We came to know about his fasting of 211 days through Dr. Laxmiben Khona and Chandrahas Khona of Ahmedabad and so we invited him in our conference to explain his aim of fasting and his feeling during fasting, "said Dr. P.G. Shah the president of Health Care International Multitherapy Institute who organised the above conference. He informed that during the First International conference on Multiple Healing Systems which was held at Ahmedabad during 4-6 December, 1998.

Hirabhai declared that he will be on fasting from 1st January 2000.

Doctors observing Shri Hira Ratan Manek:

- Dr. K.K. Shah
- Dr. P.G. Shah
- Dr. P.D. Doshi
- Dr. H.C. Mehta

- Dr. Sudhir Shah
- Dr. Viresh Patel
- Dr. Nalin Gheewala
- Dr. Hamendra Modi

"Earlier, he used to do small fasts for 10 to 20 days. But, when he completed the 211 days fast, his weight was reduced by 41 kg. and the Sugar level (Glucose) was lowered to 43. Medical Science says that when the glucose level of a human being decreasing below 50, then the situation becomes dangerous, even though in his case nothing has happend." Said Dr. P.D. Doshi the secretary of Health Care International Multitherapy Institute. Hirabhai was ready to go for continuous medical check up during his fasting from 1st January, 2000 onwards. So we took up the challenge and asked him to stay at Ahmedabad during this period. He agreed, so now we are doing medical check up jointly with Jain Doctors Federation."

After the successful completion of the fast, he was living with nine types of liquids only. Food and fruits were totally avoided. Subsequently he started dropping liquids one by one and from 1st January, 2000 he is fully fasting. He is not taking anything except water. This water will be taken only after boiling and that too from sunrise to sunset. He, who is also a member of the Solar Energy Society of India, has proved that human beings can live depending on solar energy for months together without taking any other food. He has completed 100 fasts on 9th April and he would like to study the importance of the solar energy in the human body.

"Fasting is a method of curing by meditation of mind and body which has been proved by great Jain monks, sanyasis and munis of ancient times. There is a need to propagate these methods during this age of increasing diseases of the body and mind due to overconsumption and increasing with fasting would help maintain perfection," says Dr. K.K. Shah the past president of Indian Medical Association and the present president of Jain Doctors Federation.

"Hirabhai has completed 166 fasts on 14th June, 2000 and we are very much satisfied with his health. Initially his weight was 77 kg which has now reduced up to 62 kg. All other parameters are normal. We are keeping daily record of pulse, temperature, blood pressure, water intake, urine output, weight, hours of sleep etc. Blood and Urine examination, ECG etc. are done regularly. Investigations like TC, DC, Hb, blood urea, serum creatinine, serum acetone, lipid profiles etc. are done. Solar power could sustain you for days together without food and it has now been scientifically established that all other sources of energy will get dried up sooner or later."

"I have been trying to evolve a lifestyle based on effective uses of solar energy, reduced consumption and perfect mental calm through meditation which would solve many of the problems now threatening human existence," Hirabhai said.

"The aim of fasting is to break all Karma and to achieve Moksha. But apart from that it gives your body and mind inner strength and calmness. I believe that during fasting the solar energy provides energy to the body and if you can get energy from the Sun directly you need not eat any food," says Hirabhai.

He was staying at Kachhi Jain Samaj, Paldi, Ahmedabad with free accommodation during 27th December, 1999 to 5th April, 2000. Then he was at Dr. P.D. Doshi's hospital—Sharda Hospital, Asarwa, Ahmedabad during 6th April to 6th May, 2000 with free accommodation. From 7th May he is at Shri Popatlal Doue's house. Free accommodation is given to Shri Hirabhai by Shri Popatbhai Dave and Ullasbhai Dave for which all members of Health Care International

Multitherapy Institute and Jain Doctors Federation are
very thankful to them.

Shri Hira-Ratan-Manek's current address: 2, Parag
Society, C/o, Shri Popatlal Dave, Nr. Opera Jain
Vpashrya, New Vikasgruh Road, Ahmedabad-7.

- Health Care International Multitherapy Institute:
  President : Dr. P.G. Shah, Ph.: 079-6620472.
  Secretary : Dr. P.D. Doshi, Ph.: 079-2134551
- Jain Doctors Federation:
  President : Dr. K.K. Shah, Ph.: 079-6578936
  Secretary : Dr. Himont Shah, Ph.: 079-6405201

On August 27, 2002, the following report by SHYAM
PAREKH appeared in *The Times of India*.

US Scientists Study Indian's Fasting Feat

Times News Network [Monday, August 26, 2002,
11:55:53 p.m.]

AHMEDABAD: When a 64-year-old Gujarati
mechanical engineer went without food for 411 days,
he provided some food for thought to American
scientists.

Kozhikode-based Hira Ratan Manek survived only on
boiled water and sunlight from January 1, 2000 to
February 15, 2001, causing Americans to wonder if they
could develop a technique to enable astronauts to go
without food for long periods.

Impressed by his logic-defying feat, a team of eight
US doctors and scientists, including an ophthalmologist,
a neurologist, an ayurveda expert, an acupuncture
specialist, a yoga researcher and a psychiatrist is now
examining him. Eminent neuroscientist George Brainard,
whose research on the effects of light on the human
pineal gland is funded by the National Aeronautics and
Space Administration, is also in the team. Mr. Manek was
invited to the US in June under 'Project HRM' to study

his fasting technique. The team is studying 'subtle energies' under 'Experiments with Solar, Thermal and Hydro Energetics in Human Subjects'.

Currently at Wilmington, Delaware, Mr. Manek has been fasting for more than two months and has established his genuineness, posing a challenge to conventional science and concepts about the limits of human tolerance to hunger.

"US doctors have completed the first part of the three-phase study, thoroughly examining his body with the latest equipment. The second phase of fasting is on," said city-based neuro-physician Sudhir Shah, who has been appointed advisor and consultant to the US team.

A number of volunteers are helping the US team by undertaking similar fasts under a specially-developed protocol facilitating similar studies in the US and India. A panel of 20 doctors headed by Dr. Shah had monitored Mr. Manek's fast in Ahmedabad.

The panel also included general practitioners Prakash Doshi and P.G. Shah, surgeon K.K. Shah, endocrinologist Navnit Shah and neuro-radiologist Gargeya Sutariya. They had scanned his body with magnetic resonance imaging (MRI) before and after the fast, in addition to a plethora of other tests.

"Perhaps his body is undergoing 'chronic adaptation', learning to survive on very few calories as compared to the 1,800 calories a day required for normal persons."

He said the most amazing part of Mr. Manek's feat was that he was physically active and carried on all normal activities during his fast. "On the 404th day of the fast, he climbed Palitana hill (to reach a Jain temple). And believe me, he was faster than many who were eating plenty," he said.

Subsequently, another report from a Jain website said: Hira Ratan Manek is now in America from June 18, 2002 to December 17, 2002. Currently, he is performing 109 days fasting by Jain tradition and is on a lecture tour to various cities in USA like Orlando, Los Angeles, Philadelphia, Releigh, New York, Miami, Dallas, Washington D.C., Rochester and others. The Parna (breaking of the fast) of his 109 days fasting is scheduled to be celebrated on October 27, 2002, Sunday at 10:00 A.M. at Hindu Society Hall in Orando, Florida.

CHAPTER 2

A Hypothesis on Prolonged Fasting

Dr. Navneet Shah, M.D. FICA (U.S.A.) Physician Endocrinologist, submitted the following hypothesis on July 13, 2001, on prolonged fasting to explain the Hira-Ratan-Manek phenomenon.

This is unique. You will agree that such a prolonged continuous Jain fasting for religious (the spreading of Ahimsa and other high mottos) and scientific purposes (to create awareness about Sun-energy) and also aimed at a solution of four-way human crisis (physical, mental, food and neurological) under scrupulous daily medical supervision is unheard of. It is just fantastic, and absolutely amazing, but this is not a myth. It is not happening in Himalayas or distant jungles. It is happening in Ahmedabad, Gujarat (India) in the continuous presence of the public and under strict medical check and supervision by an expert doctor team.

There is no reason to be sceptical. One may personally come and check and scrutinize. We doctors have done all these months and fellow men have been staying with him all throughout. And also several visitors see him throughout the day and night. Mr. Hira Ratan Manek has completed a 411 day fast successfully on 14th February 2001. It started from 1.1.2000. He was on total fasting as per Jainism. He was consuming boiled water daily only between 11 a.m. to 4 p.m., no other liquids and just no other food, no I/V or I/M injections. He was completely kept isolated while under strict observation.

Medical check-up commenced a few days before fasting programme and continued till today. It consists of daily written record of pulse, blood pressure, respiration, temperature, water intake, urine output, weight etc. and relevant Hematological and biochemical (basic and few advanced) tests periodically i.e., monthly or fortnightly. ECGs are taken regularly, Ultra Sonography, EEG, C-T Scan and MRI Brain have been taken at the end of one year and a team consisting of general practitioner doctors, physicians, surgeons, cardiologists, endocrinologist and a neurologist have been examining regularly and periodically from first day of fasting. Except for loss of 19 kgs weight (which is now stable with no further weight loss for 3 months), a slight reduction of pulse rate and B.P. and definite reduction of respiratory rate (from 18 it is now 10/minute) amazingly, there is no medical abnormality. Even the brain and mental capacities are absolutely normal. There are hardly any findings. He has stopped passing stool after 16th day of fasting and urine output is maintained at around 600 to 800 c.c. His blood sugar is 60 to 90. There is no acetone. The rest of the other parameters are normal.

It is just amazing. Isn't it? But how do we hypothesize it? How does science look at it? As per science, under normal circumstances of prolonging starvation, (under accidental situation or extraordinary situation,) human beings lose weight fast. First fat is utilized. Ketones appear in urine in the first week. Then proteins are burnt. Before that, the person becomes dull, lethargic and irritable, his logical reasoning fails and vital parameters fall and within 8 to 10 weeks, as per science the physical existence will be challenged. Here there is no such ill effect. How do we explain this? How does his energy mathematics work ? How is he still so intact with normal intellect, normal mental, function?

Though so far there is no solid thesis (as this is the first event in the world under medical supervision), there has to be some logical, scientific hypothesis.

It explains quite a bit, but also leaves a few questions unanswered, for all of us to further analyze. It also opens, at the same time, several new avenues for the coming time to work upon it (e.g. issue of obesity).

This hypothesis has four basic steps to explain energy-metabolic mathematics, i.e.

- Reducing calorie requirement by chronic adaptation.
- Deriving basic energy from cosmic source-chiefly, 'sun energy'.
- Utilizing the energy in an efficient way and recycling the same in his body.
- Genetically or phenotypically a different body disposition.

1. Chronic Adaptation Syndrome

As the body and the mind adapts to chronic stress in a healthier way, as compared to acute stress, similarly body's adaptation must be different to chronic fasting (beyond 30 days) as compared to acute fasting (e.g. 3 to 15 days). Nobody knows which is the exact point where body adapts chronically, but 30 days sound reasonable time though it may vary individually. This is some kind of hibernation, so to say. The routine calorie mathematics sounds logical and quite applicable to acute fasting where fats break up first, ketones appear in urine and weight loss starts; muscle mass reduces and vital functions and mental capacity may start slowing down. Thus in acute fasting, energy dissipated must come from stored sources of body to match 1:1 ratio of calorie consumption against utilization. In chronic adaptation; the metabolism of body must slow down. The body needs are reduced to the minimum.

This is possible by down regulation of cellular and receptor function. There is thus altering the energy metabolism to the lowest possible. Oxygen and water are supplied to cells as basic things. At this stage, the hunger center will become depressed, satiety center will be activated. So there will not be any feeling of hunger or food craving. It may be possible for such an individual to do routine activity with very low amount of energy or calories as 500-600 calories, to sustain cellular metabolism.

2. Deriving Energy from Cosmic Source - Solar Energy

Whatever low amount of energy, that is required, must come from some source. He is only on boiled water, which as per science as having hardly any caloric value. Or does it really supply some energy? Most likely, he is drawing energy from cosmic energy.

Cosmic Sources. Hence more correctly it is energy mathematics rather than calorie mathematics; a concept worth understanding.

Out of all cosmic sources, the SUN is the most powerful and readily available source and has been used for energy, by sages and Rishis since ancient time, including lord Mahavir, Tibetan lamas and other Rishis. Again, how is the SUN energy received? The Brain and the mind are the most powerful recipients in human body. The retina and the pineal gland (the third eye or the seat of soul as per Rene Descartes) are equipped with photoreceptor cells and may be considered photosensitive organs. As plant kingdom thrives on chlorophyll and photosynthesis, directly dependant on the Sun, similarly some photosynthesis must be taking place when we hypothesize Sun energy. Through complex ways and distinct pathways this energy must enter the body.

There is a pathway from the retinas, to the hypothalamus, called the retinohypothalamic tract. This brings information about the dark and light cycles to suprachiasmatic nucleus (SCN) of the hypothalamus. From the SCN, impulses along the nerve travel via the pineal nerve (Sympathetic nerves system) to the pineal gland. These impulses inhibit the production of Melatonin. When these impulses stop (at night or in the dark, when the light no longer stimulates the hypothalamus) pineal inhibition ceases, and Melatonin is released. The pineal gland (or the third eye) is therefore a photosensitive organ and an important timekeeper for the human body. The unexplored process of energy synthesis and transformation from the sun energy perhaps partly occurs here.

While going through the details of recent scientific literature and also comparing it with ancient Indian spiritual texts, as well as western occult and new age material the following is apparent. The activation of pineal gland is the key step in psychic, spiritual and energy transformation processes. Here in this gland, energy processing and re-distribution occurs. Pineal gland is the commander of all endocrine glands, therefore controlling the humeral system. It also regulates the circadian rhythm, sleep wake cycle and it also slows down the aging process. It has psychic properties and is the seat of soul or mind—so called third eye. It is the Agna (Ajna) chakra of tantric system. Its activation can be done with prolonged yoga and meditation techniques or through practice of solar energy. The latter does not use classic yoga steps. Pineal also inhibits growth and metastasis of some tumours. It has a stimulatory effect on the immune system. In birds and other animals, it has a magnetic material and is therefore the navigation center in birds.

Scientists are looking at magnetic, navigatory properties of pineal gland in humans. So pineal activation and charging through solar energy is the vital step and that is the doorway of energy highway. This may be Kundalini Shakti activation, in other words. Normal Pineal gland measures 6 x 8 mm in human body.

As per C.T. Scan & MRI Scan reports of Mr. Hira Ratan Manek, it is 8 x 11 mm (enlarged). This may indirectly support the important role of pineal gland in energy transformation. However, it may be mentioned that anatomically enlarged gland does not necessarily always mean hyper function.

Ever since mankind has started ignoring the psychically and Spiritually equipped pineal gland it has fallen on merely physical-material plane and endless pains have fallen on mankind. Mankind must now relearn to activate pineal and the other psycho-spiritual bodies either through cosmic energy dynamics or through practice of Rajyoga or the Tantric ways or other such practices. Kundalini Shakti is said to be activated through these and happiness and bliss with peace are bound to follow.

This light energy may be transformed into electrical, magnetic or chemical energies in body. Once processed, this energy must be transported and must be stored somewhere. Actually the ultimate form of all energy is light. Energy and light can be transformed into matter and back again to energy. Hypothalamus is the commander of autonomic nervous system and Pineal gland is in proximity to autonomic nervous system, so it is logical that new energy transportation may either activate this system or it may use this system as vehicle.

Parasympathetic nerves and its hormones and chemicals may be more useful than sympathetic system. As sympathetic system increases body needs (e.g. thinking, fighting stress, excitement etc.), para-sympathetic system is known to reduce the energy needs. It keeps the person serene and at mental peace and alters the metabolic requirements to a lower state and puts it to sleep. There may be other hormones or chemicals too. The role of temporal lobe and limbic system also may be important. It may work as a regulator if not receptor and may be psychically involved in directing the energy in proper pathways. Deep into the limbic systems or in the parts of medulla oblongata, this energy may ultimately be stored and from time to time, may be recalled, charged or recycled. Medulla oblongata has all vital centers and therefore can be proposed as store of vital energy.

Thus, there are energy receivers or receptors, processors analyzers, transformers, storers etc. to explain the energy logistics. As this form of energy mathematics is different from what we conventionally are used to in form of food and calorie mathematics; we will call this micro-food or mind utilization food (Manobhakshi Aahar). Here, we have talked about the Sun energy, but one may use any source from the cosmos, i.e. air, water, plants, earth etc. This may be called Surya vigyan, but equally there is Chandra vigyan and Vanaspati vigyan as mentioned in our ancient texts.

Also apart from retina and pineal gland, skin and other senses may be responsible for receiving the energy. In short, this opens up tremendous possibilities. This micro-food can solve the food crisis on earth and in fact is the only possible food in present context for somebody who wants to be a long-term space traveler or planet traveler. Amazing! It is time to note that our routine food is not the only source to sustain the body. The role of mind: Whatever said, in this step, (i.e. the step II of deriving the energy from the sun and transforming it in body) the mind may play the crucial role. It is well known that the mind has enormous capacity, (the soul has even further or infinite capabilities). Through Sun Tratak and Meditation, tremendous capacities are born which will bring tranquility to mind and also slow down metabolism, as mentioned in step I.

Mind can do everything including so-called miracles. It can revitalize body, it can heal diseases, it can know things in advance and it can manipulate laws of physics. It's unclear till this date whether mind is a separate entity or the pineal gland itself. The faith and blessings from Yogis and Gurus have their own roles sustaining ones self in adverse situations. On religious days, under high spirits and a cultivated atmosphere, a few people surprisingly do unusual things like walking on fire or piercing pointed swords, through their bodies without damaging themselves. If similarly, someone does fasting, these phenomena may help to pull him/her through the period of physiological problems till one enters the chronic adaptation phase.

3. Energy Economy in efficient ways and re-cycling the energy in his own body

Those who are chronically deprived of energy learn to utilize the available energy in more efficient ways—so that even at the low energy state body metabolism and vital functions including nervous system do not suffer. This is quite logical and one can imagine this happening in the individuals caught in natural calamities, or those left alone in the sea or survivors of high altitudes after plane crash etc. managing to live for several days or weeks, without food. Also, one can hypothesize that these people may be recycling the energy in their own bodies. This may be done, through complex mechanisms, involving neural and humeral organs. Solar energy, dissipated through body may get absorbed into the earth and while walking bare footed on the soil, standing in the sun, may help absorbing this energy through skin of toes, sole of feet as Shri Hira Ratan Manek does regularly and always preaches to do so to recycle the energy. This may be related to the principles of acupressure or reflexology.

4. Genetypically or phenotypically a different body predisposition

We should also examine this aspect carefully, as this leaves scope for an important discussion—whether each and every individual can use sun energy and if so, so efficiently? Only time can answer this. But it is possible that each individual has a different genetic code and also each body has different physical capabilities. Hence, one may be able to receive this Solar energy more readily, can transform and store it in a better way and also can utilize more efficiently and even recycle it—while another person may not be able to do it to the same extent. Hence, experiments, must be taken up, if possible on a randomized base upon volunteers with control population. However, leaving this component aside for the time being, it is possible that many people can do this experiment very successfully under supervision. Prior body checkup and particularly retinal-ophthalmic checkup is mandatory and under strict medical guidance, a graded time bound experiment upon volunteers may be taken up.

If this theory can be generalized, then it can change the destiny of mankind. First of all, the food crisis will be solved. Through activation of this supreme energy in body and transforming it into electrical, chemical and magnetic forms, people can not only become free of diseases but can gain positive health with a vibrant aura. His luster can impress even enemies; the enmity may dissolve. With improvement of mental and intellectual capacities one may be able to use brain power up to 90 to 100 %, as against to 3 - 10% as we normally do. There will be a reign of peace and prosperity. As there is no food, the bad thoughts and ill feelings will be stopped, so eternal peace is bound to follow.

This will also question the routine common calorie mathematics. By this, there is a challenge to the routine calorie based science. Its limitations are highlighted, at the same time the complex issues of obesity and malnutrition can be readily explained through the concept of solar energy. It is possible that obese people, though not eating excess food, still receive energy from cosmic sources explaining their obesity. The concept of cosmic energy can be used thus for total uplift of mankind at physical, mental, intellectual, supramental and spiritual levels. Extensive scientific research work therefore should be immediately taken up, by appropriate authorities, including bioscientists and medical personnel, to answer all these issues.

(Ref. case study of Mr. Hira Ratan Manek : 411 fast : 375 fast completed on 9-1-2001.)

Dr. Sudhir V. Shah M.D., D.M. Neurophysician 206-8, Sangini Complex, Nr. Parimal Crossing, Ellisbridge, Ahmedabad-380 006. Ph. : (c) 079-646 70 52 (R) 079-662 17 42. Hon. Neurologist : H.E. The Governor of Gujarat, India. President : Asso. of Physician of A'bad. (97-98) Hon. Asst.Prof. of neurology : Sheth K.M School of PGMR Smt. N.H.L. M.M College Hon. Neurologist: V.S.Hospital, Ahmedabad. Jivraj Mehta Smarak Hospital. I acknowledge suggestions and help received for this hypothesis. From : (1) Dr. Navneet Shah M.D. FICA (U.S.A.) Physician Endocrinologist (C) 6425566. (2) Dr. Gargey Sutaria (M.D.) & Dr. Kalpesh Shah (M.D.) Radiologist Usmanpura C.T.Scan Centre. Clinical Assistant: Dr. Nalin Gheewala M.D. Physician. Dr. K.K. Shah M.S. Surgeon. Dr. Viresh Patel M.D. Physician. Dr. P.G. Shah M.B.B.S. Family Physician. Dr. P.D. Doshi M.B.B.S. Family Physician.

CHAPTER 3

Prana-Mystery Building Stone
of the Universe

Gerd Lange, Co-director, In-Breath, provides his experience of Living on Light in the context of his knowledge of prana.

What Indian sages thousands of years ago called "prana", the ancient Chinese named "chi" or "ki" and the Druids refer to as "od" or "id". It is commonly agreed, that prana is the life force but too small or etheric to be perceived by any kind of instrument or measuring device to date.

Modern science has found that our seemingly so solid world vibrates in an eternal dance of swirling atoms. These in turn consist of even smaller and smaller particles, which finally turn out to be pure energy (prana) densified in various wavelets and aggregates to form matter. In general, there are two things which we take in when we breathe. One is air and the other is prana, pure life-force energy itself, more vital than air for our existence. If you take away air, you have a couple of minutes before you die; if you take away water, you have even more time; and if you take away food you have much more time still, but if you break prana from spirit, death is instantaneous. So taking in prana with breath is absolutely crucial in sustaining our life. Prana is not just in the air, it is everywhere. There is nowhere that it is not; it even exists in a vacuum or a void. Nothing exists without prana, neither animate nor inanimate. Prana is the smallest, most refined, miniature building block of life, subtlest of subtle energies which creates and sustains simply everything (physical matter, thoughts, feelings, etc.). Prana in my opinion is higher dimensional creative energy and inseparably connected to spirit, god or creative energy.

I have always been interested in Prana and its spiritual capacity. Being a Rebirther for many years, I have discovered, that the amazing effects which I continuously witness in a "breath", simply can't be produced just by the oxygen content accumulated in the session or through my guidance alone. There always seems to be an inner intelligence at work which undeniably suggests to me a connection with the Divine.

So what actually happens during a breathing session? We humans are an intricately layered four body energy system, consisting of a physical, emotional, mental and spiritual body—made of prana in various states of densification (i.e. wavelengths or vibrational harmonies). Each of these bodies is an electromagnetic energy field in form of a grid system, which resonates, in a specific frequency, not unlike an electronic computer memory bank. Each of these bodies functions on a different level and performs vital life interactions, e.g. processes information, holds memory and performs a multitude of other functions. The four bodies are linked through the chakra system.

If unaligned (through shock, trauma, emotions) the mesh of these grids collects densified subtle energies (unreleased feelings, dysfunctional thought patterns, etc.) instead of letting them pass through. These unprocessed energies get trapped in the system. Moving through the layers, thoughts densify into emotions, emotions densify into physical sensations and finally solidify in physical symptoms—disease and illness.

Breathing intentionally, in a conscious connected manner, increases the prana content in the four layers of the grid systems. Accumulating prana in the bodies helps to realign the grids by energising them, which raises their vibrational frequencies. This in turn entices all four grid systems simultaneously to resonate in a higher frequency and they automatically attempt to achieve a state of unity, a place of balance. Through the realignment the trapped densified energies loosen up, and get "washed out" by the free floating prana, to be transported to the electromagnetic surface (consciousness). There it is processed by re-experiencing and released as thought, emotion or sensation. This leaves your system more cleansed, realigned and connected.

As we have established a few paragraphs back, prana is in everything and everything consists of it. God (Source, the creative principle) per definition also is everything and everything consists of and through him/her/it . Therefore, it seems clear to me that prana must be of divine nature and has to have a direct connection to Source. As prana is pure spirit, the "breather" usually connects to Source in a breathing session via the spiritual body. Experiences include feeling warm and internally glowing, cared for and loved, mystical revelations and unity consciousness during the integration phase. Another fascinating by-product of this breathing technique is that it facilitates permanent Higher Self-connection. Initially, you just get in touch with your Higher Self but over time you can establish a permanent conscious connection to your inner knowing, the Divine One Within (DOW) and your true nature as soul having a human experience.

Newest information suggest that once upon a time we actually were consciously and continuously connected to the infinite supply of prana and existed purely of it. Not too long ago—about 13,000 years, before the last poleshift erased our conscious memory of it, we used to breathe in such a way, that while air came in through our mouth and nose, we would take prana in through the top of our heads—what once was the soft spot on the top of our heads. Simultaneously, we took the prana in from below, through the perineum. If you carefully observe how new-born babies breathe you can actually observe this—a gentle pulsation at the fontnelle and the perineum. The prana channel goes through the body like a vertical axle and is about two inches in diameter. It extends one hand length above the head and one hand length below the feet and connects with the crystalline energy field (Mer-Ka-Ba) around the body. The prana then flows in from above and below the body and meets in one of the chakras. The chakra in which the prana meets depends on where you are mentally, emotionally, and dimensionally "tuned."

After the poles shifted, we stopped breathing in this manner and started taking in the prana through our mouth and nose directly with the air. The prana then bypassed the pineal gland in the centre of the head. The pineal gland is an eye—the third eye—not the pituitary gland as often thought of. It is shaped like an eyeball, round, hollow, with a lens for focusing light and colour receptors. It is designed to receive light from above to go to every cell in the body instantaneously. Normally this gland should be about the size of a quarter but in us it has become the size of a pea because we haven't used it for about 13,000 years.

The direct result of turning off the pineal gland is polarity consciousness—good and bad, right and wrong. Because of the way we breathe we see things in terms of good and evil, but in fact Unity is all there is; there is just one God and one Spirit that moves through everything.

When I met Jasmuheen, two-and-a-half years ago, at an international conference for Breathworkers (GIC) things got really interesting for me. She gave a lecture there, about the possibility of being able to live without eating, living on light, purely being sustained by prana (which was the way we existed in the times when we utilised the prana tube). All you had to do is to connect to the Divine One Within (DOW) and to allow yourself to be fed by it through an alternative source of nourishment, the most refined, most pure form of energy, by God him/herself, by prana.

This genuinely blew my mind, especially as my immediate, internal reaction was a huge YES!!!. Actually being quite fond of eating and cooking, with a rather strong tendency to overeating, I was surprised at having had such a reaction. But over time and through my growing involvement with her example (and that of thousands of other people having done this 21-day reprogramming process successfully in the meanwhile) it became very clear to me that living on prana is a true and mind-expanding possibility. Being able to be sustained on energy alone would mean to me the definite proof that I am a light being, that I am not the body, but something much more refined and expanded. I had always intuitively known and felt this, but there hadn't been any definite proof so far. Her theory, however outrageous it was, made total sense to me. Based on the information of the prana tube, my firm belief that prana was everything and of divine nature and my strong connection to my DOW simply urged me to give this possibility a try.

The good news was that, if properly prepared and trusting, anyone could do the 21-day process. You didn't have to be a saint, which would have definitely counted me out. The biggest challenge for me now was to actually find a month of free time in my absolutely busy schedule. I had to wait for nearly 2 years before my chance had come. In hindsight of course this waiting period was very valuable, as it gave me the opportunity to research in more depth and to speak with lots of people who had done the process already. Through their reports and experiences I reached a place of knowing in me, beyond any trace of doubt, that it is truly possible to live on light, to live on prana.

My partner Yamini, who had also met Jasmuheen at this conference and had the same reaction as me, found time to do her process two months before me. Seeing her going through the process with all its challenges, but coming out of it renewed and changed in a more empowered, grounded way, inspired me even further. Then finally my time had come too. I won't go into details of the process here as there is not enough time and space for it right now, but it was an amazing, yet ordinary time. I feel totally changed, yet curiously the same. A definite transition has happened to me, including a complete realignment of my body and physical structure, and yet I feel "it's still me", just with a difference. The most obvious difference of course is, that I don't have to eat anymore.

For me it is now over 160 days (5 months+) since I stopped having to eat and Yamini is over the 200 days mark by now. Our weight has stabilised, our energy levels are high and we fully participate in life. Yamini is working out regularly at the gym, whereas I, of course, still have no time for that as usual (working some days up to 16 hours). By now our initial thoughts of "did it really work?" have been totally removed. We both know for certain, we are fully sustained by pranic energy alone—which is amazing. Somehow a miracle and yet it seems quite nomal and ordinary to us.

I am comparing the process (and the fact that we don't need to eat anymore) to an enormous fire walk. You can only do it safely when you absolutely know that you can. If you have any doubt about it, you will burn your feet and its the same with the process. As long as you have doubt and disbelief it will be impossible for you to do it. This seems total proof to me that thought is creative, that we are consciously creating our reality at any given time, and that there are amazing possibilities out there which we haven't explored yet.

As we have established beforehand, prana is of electromagnetic nature. This suggests that it is possible to charge and program prana with your intentional thought energy and that you can use it for conscious creation and healing, for yourself and for the highest good of this planet and its people. So if you are interested in global issues and want to make a definite contribution start breathing in love and light and breathe out love, peace, compassion and positive intentions for the highest in humanity. Create your own reality, your own vision version of paradise on earth, and radiate out your personal (and hopefully) positive charge of that.

CHAPTER 4

Breatharianism: The Secret You've been Looking for !

Ahmen Heaven here gives his impressions of Breatharianism and one of its early practitioners:

"I'm not against eating...I'm not against MacDonald hamburgers...I'm not against the establishment...I'm not against anything...and...I'm not looking for any followers."—Wiley Brooks. I had read about "breatharians" (people who live without eating) in a few esoteric health books, but never considered it a possibility for myself, or for any modern man or woman in the western world. Then I heard about Wiley Brooks, a self-proclaimed breatharian, who made national news in the late 70's, claiming that he had been living without eating for about twenty years.

Brooks, who was 50-year old at the time, came to Hawaii in 1983 to give a talk and then a 3-day seminar. I attended both. Besides the subject matter, I was very impressed by his deep penetrating voice, his ability to stay calm, centered, relaxed, and focused, even under hostile questioning from the audience, and by his obviously limber and lithe body for a man of his age.

I came to the 3-day "breatharian" seminar in Hawaii, but without the $300 fee to attend. Wiley asked me: "If you can't find $300, then how do you expect to find God?"

Within 15 minutes, I had the $300. At first, I was the

biggest skeptic, and prodded Wiley at every opportunity, trying to find fault wherever I could. I forgot the saying: "As you seek, so shall you find." Since I had been looking for error, I found it wherever I could. However, had I been seeking for the truth, I would have found plenty of that as well. Finally, after a couple of days at the seminar, I was converted, at least in my beliefs if not actions. I became convinced that Wiley was telling the truth, and that "breatharianism" is a revolutionary and important concept. As Wiley says: "They laughed at the Wright brothers... and they ridiculed Thomas Edison..." Wiley Brooks is an intelligent human being with much goodness in his heart, and wants to help people experience an increased sense of well-being and joy, which comes from not-eating, rather than eating as we have been told.

Later that year, Wiley was caught in a scandal. The newspaper headline read: "Breatharian caught eating." It seemed so interesting and comical that it made local papers all over the U.S. and even the national news.

Wiley simply denies the story entirely, and I think he may have staged the whole event so as to keep himself from being thrown in a nut-house. What happened was that his lady friend (lover and business partner), with whom he had just broken off a romantic relationship, claimed that she saw Wiley sneaking into a "7-11" late at night, to buy some twinkies! There are several variations to the same story—although it is hard to believe any of them, since I have actually met Wiley and spent 3 or 4 days with him, as well as spoken with him, and listened to him, for many hours. I am not here to prove breatharianism, or to disprove it, only to establish the truth. (Wiley denies the whole story about the twinkies at 7-11, and claims that his ex-lover/business partner made up the whole story just to discredit him, because he had just broken off his romantic relationship with her).

The thing about breatharianism, which Wiley emphasizes, is that it is a way to great happiness, as well as to physical well-being. From my own personal experience, as well as from observation of others, I am convinced that "fasting" (in general) is good for one's health and happiness, and not just for losing weight.

I have found that really great happiness, as well as exceptional mental clarity, and even increased sex drive, comes from fasting, rather than from eating.

Arnold Ehret (author of *"Rational Fasting"* and *"Mucusless Diet Healing"*), who did many public fasts in the latter 1800's and early 1900's, also noted his rapid hair growth during fasts. Dr. Ronald Klatz, President of the American Academy of Anti-Aging Medicine, and author of *"Grow Young with HGH"* (i.e., Human Growth Hormone) (published 1997) also notes that one of the human actions that will increase the secretion of human growth hormone (HGH), is fasting from food. HGH is considered rejuvenative, and many people are spending thousands of dollars a month taking HGH supplements or injections... The same effect can come naturally, from fasting.

Wiley has explained many times how he "discovered" breatharianism through numerous experiences with fasting, in the 1960s: "Every time I fasted, I felt great... My mind became clear, and I got stronger, felt lighter, younger, and healthier... but whenever I went back to eating, my mind got less clear, I got tired, and all the old symptoms returned again."

Wiley admits that everybody is not going to be a breatharian, and that most people aren't even interested. He also says that he "doesn't care if anybody is interested or not interested"... "But for those people who ARE interested, in being healthy and happy, then breatharianism can certainly help you get there in a hurry. It is very FAST and very EFFICIENT."

Wiley is not a dogmatist, which is another attraction. He suggests that any way we can purify our blood, we should use that method, but he also adds that he has been looking for a better system than his, 24 hours a day, and that if he hasn't found it by now, it just doesn't exist.

Wiley says that he sleeps about one hour a night, or just one night a week. He relates sleeping and eating.

The more you eat, the more you must sleep. As we already spend a third of our entire lives in sleep, this appears to be a way to significantly lengthen our waking lives.

A day or several days spent in fasting, seems to take a long time, while there is abundant mental energy for meditation, introspection, and prayer.

Fasting, then, seems to make time last longer, and increases the time available to experience more, as well as improves our ability to appreciate it all.

What does Wiley do then, if he doesn't eat or sleep? Does he ever get bored? Wiley says: "I assure you, there is nothing boring about being a breatharian. There are thousands of things to do."

"You can eat if you want to; that's your prerogative... I used to play that game... I know what it's like... But I'm just not interested in it any more... I'm not interested in going out, and working for the money to buy the food, then shopping for it, then going home and preparing it, then eating it, then washing the dishes, then just letting it all out in the toilet... and in the end, you end up in a box, in the ground, on the outside of town." Meanwhile, we can't figure out why we don't feel that good, or why we don't have enough energy (another reason many people mistakenly eat more), or why we don't look that good... and we spend billions of dollars annually on ways to lose weight. In the Bible, even Jesus reminds us that "Food goes into the belly, and is cast out into the sewer."

Wiley admits to eating on a number of occasions, in the first 20 years after he became a breatharian. But he says that the food left him feeling sick every time, and obviously did not sustain him, or give him life.

Wiley says: "Life comes only from life, and there is only one source of life, which is God." But he says " these liquids and solids, which we call food, do not give us life, or health, or beauty," as we are programmed to believe by the food industry.

The food-industry is the largest industry in the world, but it is unlikely that "breatharianism" will ever put a dent in food-industry profits, since eating is such an intrinsic aspect of society, as well as an addictive and accepted, pleasurable behavior (although it is also accompanied by a lot of pain).

What may happen, however, is that there is a possibility that there might come a time in the foreseeable future when there just isn't any food to eat. "The food supply on the planet is getting less and less, and the quality is getting worse and worse... It would be wise to look into breatharianism, just in case you are ever confronted with a time when you don't have any food to eat." (Wiley suggests that the best thing to do in such a situation is to empty your intestinal tract, rather than fight over any remaining food.)

Wiley does not recommend jumping into breatharianism immediately, but he does suggest that we should rejoice just knowing that purification of the blood is the secret to health, happiness, and long life... "This is the secret you've been looking for."

Wiley is not the first or only breatharian. There are a number of cases of people who have lived without eating. One of the most famous, and most well-documented case of a breatharian, was Terese Neumann, a German nun, who did not eat anything at all for 35 years, between 1922 and 1957. There are at least seven books about her life. One of the best of these books is by an author named Johann Steiner. In these books, several other cases of "food abstainers" are referred to, and the one trait they all had in common was that they all had the uncommon gift of clairvoyance. (Even Wiley claims to be psychic, and able to see into the future).

For all these reasons, I find nothing objectionable, or extraordinary, or incredulible, about breatharianism. After all, it has been estimated that about 10% of all teenage girls in America are anorexic. Wiley says: "It doesn't take any discipline to be a breatharian... all it takes is understanding...It doesn't take any discipline to keep from standing in the middle of the road when cars are passing by... and I can assure you, that when you UNDERSTAND that the food you are eating is NOT giving you life and vitality, with increased energy, health and happiness, it won't take any discipline to STOP taking it."

"Breatharianism is just a simple understanding of how the human body works." Then someone asked him what is the purpose of the alimentary canal. "The purpose of the alimentary canal is to get rid of wastes from the body." Even Wiley admitted to going to the toilet every few months, proving the usefulness of this organ.

"But if food is so good for you, how come the body keeps trying to get rid of it?... Man was not designed to be a garbage can like he is." Wiley says he sees "a lot of people who are waiting to get their happiness in heaven, but meanwhile are suffering like hell, here on earth."

CHAPTER 5

What is Living on Light?

Here Jasmuheen answers some basic questions:

"Breatharian" refers to those who choose to neither eat nor drink, who obtain nourishment from the universal life force—prana—directly, much in the way Indian yogis are nourished when "buried alive." The term prana signifies both the cosmic life energy and its subtle biological conductor in the body and the two are inseparable. It pervades each cell, like electricity through atoms in a battery. Its biological counterpart, apana, is a fine essence residing in the brain and nervous system, capable of generating a subtle radiation impossible to analyze in a laboratory, which circulates in the organism as motor impulse and sensation.

In *Kundalini, the Evolutionary Energy in Man*, Gopi Krishna writes: "All systems of Yoga are based on the supposition that living bodies owe their existence to the agency of an extremely subtle immaterial substance, pervading the universe and designated as prana, which is the cause of all organic phenomena, controlling the organisms by means of the nervous system and brain, manifesting itself as the vital energy.

The prana, in modern terminology 'vital energy,' assumes different aspects to discharge different functions in the body and circulates in the system in two separate streams, one with fervid and the other with frigid effect, clearly perceptible to yogis in the 'awakened condition'.

Understanding prana as the essence of life, we can see how an organism can be sustained by the etheric realms and prana alone. Individuals who have achieved this are called breatharians.

Living on Light is a less rigid program, where one may choose to exist on liquid light but still drink for pleasure and taste sensation. The 21-day initiation process is not one of denial or fasting towards ascension. It is one of mastery, a sacred, spiritual journey being pioneered to present to humanity (and the Western world) another option. One can be vegetarian, vegan, fruitarian, liquidarian or breatharian. Not a miracle, or something to be feared, it is a reclamation of our natural state of being. When one ceases to require physical nourishment from food the energy used in the digestive process can be redirected. The benefits are numerous, and as each individual is unique so is each experience. Ancient spiritual teachings speak of the "in breath" and "out breath" of God. Our journey home is the in breath, the journey into light. As we refine our frequency, and embrace the "God I Am" more completely, there must come a point where we are sustained once more by the essence of that which we are.

CHAPTER 6

Those in 'BIGU' State
Don't Go Hungry

Practitioners of qigong live comfortably on 300 calories
a day or less according to Caroline Terenzini of *Centre
Daily Times*. She writes:

An average adult eats 2,000 or more calories a day, but
some practitioners of a Chinese meditative discipline
called qigong have achieved a state that lets them live
comfortably on 300 calories a day or less. Some
practitioners report maintaining the bigu (pronounced
bee-goo) state for years.

Yi Fang, a Penn State researcher and coordinator of a
conference at Penn State that explored qigong and bigu
from a scientific perspective, compared bigu to the
superconducting phenomenon in materials science. "It
is hard to believe," Fang acknowledged. "The scientific
community sees it as a violation of energy conservation
laws and others say it isn't normal." But, he said, nearly
100 of the qigong practitioners attending the conference
had experienced the bigu state, and a dozen reported
they had not eaten solid food for five or more years.

Draconian as that sounds, people who achieve bigu
are able to maintain a healthy weight and to follow their
daily routines without discomfort or fatigue, said Fang,
47, who is a research associate at Penn State's Materials
Research Laboratory.

A practitioner for 17 years, Fang said over the past seven years he has generally eaten only one meal a day, with no animal products. During that time, he has achieved the bigu state occasionally for several weeks at a time. During bigu, which can be translated as "living on light," Fang said, he is able to live comfortably on about 300 calories a day, generally from fruit juices.

"You do not experience hunger," he said. Indeed, he added, eating unneeded food takes time and energy. While an overweight person might lose weight in the bigu state, the 5-foot-5 Fang said he stays close to his usual 110 pounds.

He described bigu as a naturally occurring phenomenon that produces a special physiological state in which the individual's blood chemistry differs from that of a person who is fasting.

"We don't force ourselves," he said. "If you force yourself, your physiology will not let you." Blood sugar will drop and the individual will be tired and hungry, he said. Instead, in bigu, a practitioner becomes "more and more efficient," Fang said, "like a super-efficient car that is able to go 250 miles on 1 gallon of gas."

For him, qigong practice has meant fewer colds and disappearance of his allergy to pollen. Fang defined qigong (pronounced chee-gung) as "a practice, a technique, a skill to improve your potential" and said its basic purpose is "to improve health and everything else follows."

"After practice, you feel more and more energetic, but your mind is calmer," he said. An ancient practice, qigong took on new life in China in the 1980s when the government relaxed strictures on such practices. Now, Fang estimates, about 10 percent of the 1.2 billion Chinese follow the discipline, which also is popular in Japan and Korea.

Fang attends two group practices a week at the Materials Research Laboratory and on other days spends up to an hour on qigong.

No Expectations

For qigong practice, participants sit forward on a chair with their feet flat on the floor, hands held palms up in front of the abdomen. Sitting quietly, they breathe deeply while listening to an audiotape that emphasizes visualization. Qigong does not require strenuous postures. "I was immediately fascinated," said Laurie Schoonhoven of State College, who tried a variety of meditative techniques before becoming a qigong practitioner last year. "It has had a profound effect on my life. It has provided an inner core of calm and balance that I never had before."

Now she practices for 15 or 20 minutes daily, mentally going over the steps. "It's sort of like a diet or exercise," she said. "If you do it once a week, it won't have any effect. You need to do it daily."

Achieving the bigu state used to be a goal, Schoonhoven said, "but now if it happens, it happens." Qigong emphasizes "no expectations," she added.

Yu Wen, 32, who is writing her dissertation for a doctorate in biology from Penn State, has been practicing qigong about five years, and in that time, she said, has experienced bigu three times, lasting one to two weeks each time.

"It was very beautiful," she said. "It's very special." During her bigu experience, said Wen, who now lives in New Jersey, she drank only fruit juice or water. "I didn't feel any different in the stomach," she noted. "I didn't feel empty. I had enough energy." "I cannot explain it," she added, "but it naturally comes, naturally goes."

Rustum Roy, founding director of the Materials Research Laboratory and chairman for the conference, has joined forces with Dr. Andrew Weil, director of a program in integrative medicine at the University of Arizona, Tucson, to form an organization to evaluate a variety of therapies, including qigong.

The purpose of Friends of Health, based in Washington, D.C., is not to validate any one practice, but "to say 'look,' " Roy said, adding: "A lot of science is not checked out. If something is bogus there, it'll come out."

Some scientific studies that have found health benefits in calorie restriction. At the University of Wisconsin, experiments with mice showed rodents that ate less lived longer, and at the Massachusetts Institute of Technology, studies of yeast metabolism, which is similar to animal metabolism, found that yeast on a low-calorie diet lived longer.

In a long-term study at the National Institute of Aging, researchers have found that rhesus monkeys fed 30 percent fewer calories than normal developed metabolic patterns indicating the animals would be more resistant to diabetes and heart disease.

Researchers caution that any such diet requires careful attention to necessary nutrients.

CHAPTER 7

Bigu and Weight Loss:
Qi as a Food Source

Dr. Qizhi Gao reports on research on Qi:

In the medical literature, obesity is referred to as a "multifactorial disorder." Defined by the National Institutes of Health as a body weight 20 percent or more above "desirable" weight, more than one-third of adult Americans are overweight. Perched at the center of chronic disease risk and psychosocial disability for millions of Americans, successful management of obesity offers unique patient care and public health opportunities. If all Americans were to achieve a normal body weight, it has been estimated that there would be a three-year increase in life expectancy, 25 percent less coronary heart disease, and 35 percent less congestive heart failure and stroke.

Unfortunately, obesity is also one of the most difficult and frustrating disorders to manage successfully. Primary care providers and patients with little benefit expend considerable effort. Using standard treatments in university settings, only 20 percent of patients lose 20 pounds at two-year follow-up, while only 5 percent of patients lose 40 pounds. This lack of clinical success has created a never-ending demand for new weight loss treatments.

A truly comprehensive programme for weight loss

mainly includes three parts: reducing caloric intake, exercise and behavior modification. The key point is reducing caloric intake, because change in weight equals caloric intake minus caloric output, according to the first law of thermodynamics. Normally, the purpose of exercise is to increase the caloric output and the purpose of behavior modification is to limit the caloric intake with self-control.

Based on the above understanding, Bigu Qigong shows its big advantage in weight loss. Bigu translates literally as "avoid (bi) the grain (gu)." In practice, it reflects the ability to live solely on qi without food.

Bigu is a period during which the qigong practitioner's vital energy transitions from the air one breathes and the essence of food and water to drawing one's sustenance strictly from the qi in the air. For the experienced qigong practitioner, this is a natural process that occurs when the accumulation of qi reaches a certain level. The ability to sustain normal body functions from qi only is possible with no change in one's daily routine and has no side effects.

Some qigong practitioners can live on the qi without food for a long period of time and oftentimes for achieving and sustaining a much higher energy level through the physical and mental discipline of the bigu exercise. For weight loss, it combines reducing caloric intake, exercise and behavior modification altogether.

One of the most elusive principles of Qigong is quantifying Qi as a vital force. Scientific methods are just beginning to define its nature, objectively supporting what has been experienced very profoundly on a more personal, subjective level. From the broadest viewpoint, everything is a form of energy.

Body energy has an anatomy and physiology uniquely its own — separate from the physical body. Despite the basic difference of air and food in terms of vibratory function and complexity, there is a homeostatic relationship between them, in which one acts as a back-up system for the other.

Bigu can be found in many ancient Chinese texts, in individual legend and exercise methods to experience. Here are a few examples: A story from Bao Puzi's Inner Treaties said that: A man name Jian was hunting in the field when he fell into a deep tomb in his early age. He was so hungry. Then he saw a big turtle, its head moved up and down to swallow the air. Jian was told that a turtle is good at Daoyin. Conducting Qi, he imitated the turtle's movement. He did not feel hungry any more until someone saved him 100 days later. After that he had the Bigu ability — living on the air without food. The emperor Wei did not believe this and placed Jian in a room without food. One year later, Jian still was full of energy and his face had a normal healthy color.

Wang Chong Lun Heng—Dao Xue Pian from the Eastern Han dynasty, stated: "The people who live on Qi have longevity, although they do not eat enough grain they are still full of energy."

Among the historical relics unearthed from the Han Tomb No. 3 at Mawangdui, Changsha, Hunan Province, there was a silk book, On Abandoning Food and Living on Qi, and a silk painting, Daoyin Illustrations, of the early Western Han Dynasty period (3rd century B.C.). The former is a method of "inducing, promoting and conducting Qi"; the latter displays 44 colored "Daoyin Illustrations in which training exercises are painted."

As a qigong practitioner, I have personally experienced Bigu twice. From July 20, 1993, until August 3, 1993, my daily diet consisted of a cup of juice or an orange. The first three days were the most difficult as I continued to feel hungry. After the three-day adjustment period, I was able to control my appetite and hunger with the qigong exercise and gradually increased my energy level, as well.

During the two-week period, I continued my normal work routine and required less sleep than normal; physically and mentally, I felt very comfortable and relaxed.

I lost a total of 10 pounds in two weeks and have never gained the weight back. I repeated the same process for a two-week period in 1996, with similar results. In June of 1996 I conducted a two-week weight loss experiment with 12 subjects, most of whom had no previous qigong experience. Subjects were initially taught two different Qigong exercises: one to control appetite and one to increase energy level. These exercises facilitated the body switching its primary nutrient source from food to Qi. Each subject was encouraged to eat and drink only what the body required. Emphasis was placed on the fact that this was not a deprivation study, rather a study to demonstrate the body's ability to derive sustenance from sources other than food and in the process promote weight reduction.

At the conclusion of the two-week study, there was a significant mean weight loss of 11.2 pounds; mean weight loss per day was 9 pounds. Energy levels gradually increased during the two-week period with a concomitant reduction of hunger. Food consumption was rated on a six-point scale, with a six representing three complete meals. Mean food consumption was rated fewer than two for all days except Day 3 and Day 11.

There was a significant increase in energy levels post exercise for nine of the 13 days (67 percent). Hunger levels were significantly reduced 10 of 13 days (77 percent). Blood pressure did not significantly change between pre-and post-measures.

Ten of the 12 subjects lost a minimum of nine pounds during the 14-day experiment; the two subjects who lost less than nine pounds (3 and 4 respectively), both performed the exercises less frequently and had a higher food consumption. All subjects returned to normal eating habits within three days of terminating the exercise. The results were presented at the Third World Conference on Medical Qigong.

Bigu qigong is a safe and effective method for weight loss that uses self-control and the exercise to reduce caloric intake; however, for the lay practitioner, it is necessary to have an experienced qigong teacher as a guide.

Bigu is a viable protocol for long-term, sustained weight loss.

Dr. Qizhi Gao is president and founder of the Kansas College of Chinese Medicine in Wichita, Kan., and is a Qigong Practitioner and Instructor.

(This article was published in its entirety by Kung Fu/ Qigong Magazine, November 1998, and was presented at the Second World Congress on Qigong, San Francisco, California, November 1997.)

CHAPTER 8

Yan Xin Qigong

There are few known cases in Yan Xin Qigong. On March 28, 1999 Dr. Yan Xin gave a qi-emitting lecture in LA. During the first half of it he spoke extensively about bigu, which is Chinese Qigong term for "living on light" or "being breatharian".

Among other things: He spoke about women in bigu—that some stop menstruating, and yet are able to conceive. (Those are the ones who wanted children). He spoke about one such a couple. They were in bigu when they conceived their child (about 4-5 years ago).

She was in bigu during the whole pregnancy. The parents still remain in "nonstandard bigu" (meaning that they take small amounts of liquids and food on occasion). He said that the child remains in nonstandard bigu too. The boy has never eaten solid food. He can consume only small amounts of liquids, otherwise, he gets "diarrhea". Other than that, the child is healthy and is developing well.

He said that the reason he was in North America at the time was to complete an 88-day study on bigu for the aerospace institute. He said that since the study was just finished and not yet published, he was not at liberty to speak of it "officially" and disclose the details. He said that since 1991 when he first came to the US and gave a series of qi-emitting lectures in the Universities of North America, hundreds of attendees experienced the bigu phenomenon. He pointed out that the big difference between bigu and fasting is that there is no feeling of hunger whatsoever. Quite the opposite, people in bigu feel more energetic than usual, sleepless and are in high spirits. Experience starts on its own accord: without premeditation or intention, one simply does not feel like eating.

He said that in 1994 there was a strong movement opposing qigong, and because of that, on many occasions he urged his audiences to come out of bigu and not to discuss this issue with the "uninitiated"—in order to avoid the controversy. Now, he said, the atmosphere is more benevolent, but still, he said that he does not encourage anyone to purposefully seek the experience. (Nonetheless, a number of people who attended the lecture on March 28, 1999 "fell" into weeks-long bigu afterwards.)

He spoke a lot about one of the IYXQA key members, who has been in bigu for 8 years. It so happened that she fainted on that day, in Illinois, just when he started the lecture in LA. The call came in and he had to attend to this emergency. He returned and described the situation. Then he laughed, "Some people here in the audience think that she must be very hungry, if she did not eat for 8 years!" "But still, please pause to consider," he continued, "This is the first time she fainted — in 8 years!" He attributed her fainting spell to her very hectic schedule and enormous drive. (The woman does not sleep either).

"I told her many times to slow down," he said, "but she would not listen. When you gotta rest, you gotta rest."

CHAPTER 9

Body Changes,
Thinking and Destiny

Harold Percival here discusses the physiology of nutrition through the breath:

What happens to certain aspects of the body when you stop to eat....The blood gradually ceases to build and maintain the body. It acts as a conveyer of nerve force. Nutrition is taken in by the breath directly from the four stages of matter by condensation. The brain takes and sends impressions more easily than was possible before. The spinal cord assumes more and more the appearance of brain structure. Its central canal becomes large, and the terminal filament, which is now atrophied from disuse is greatly enlarged. Its central canal, which at present is threadlike and is lost on its way to the end of the filament, is widened and reaches to the very tip of the filament. The intestinal tract ceases to be a feeding tube and a sewer, and the anus disappears.

The stomach and small intestines are the superfluous and disappear. The large bowel or colon, then serving a new purpose, becomes part of the nerve structure, similar to the spinal cord, termed the front-or-nature-cord. This cord with its lateral branches is made up of the former esophagus, of the two cords and the plexuses and the increased ramification of the involuntary nerve system, and of the colon. The middle of the three bands that extend along the exterior wall of the colon, becomes hollowed out, and around this canal is arranged the colon, greatly reduced in size, so that only a short, narrow tubular cord remains, as part of the front-cord.

Included in the front-cord are the right and left vagus nerves, with their ramifications. It is situated in front of the abdominal cavity and is curved backward, pointing toward the tip of the terminal filament of the voluntary nerve system.

The front-cord becomes enclosed in a resilient structure, here termed the front-or nature-cord. This replaces the sternum and is extended to and is continuous with the greatly changed pelvic bowl. The body is thus becomes a two-columned organism.

There are other changes in the body in addition to those given, which will obtain when the human enters the life path. Nerves not now visible will become active and will affect chiefly the lungs and heart. The lungs will then become more like the cerebrum, and the heart with the aorta, the thymus and other glands, like the cerebellum and pons.

CHAPTER 10

Healing with Light

The advanced medical technology of healing with light is discussed by Matt DeBow:

Light is one the most important dynamics for life. Its power and significance is just beginning to be understood. Light is energy our bodies use, its biochemical action effects the metabolic hormones in our bodies. Research has proven that to be healthy we need a certain amount light everyday. There are cases of light deficiency syndrome known as SAD (Seasonal Affective Disorder) occurring from the lack of sunlight. Light effects different enzymatic reactions, babies that suffer from jaundice are placed under blue light to help them.

As strange as it may seem pure white sun rays are actuality a composite of many colours of light. Rainbows show us the full range of color that is visible to the naked eye. Monochromatic light in scientific terms is light that has been isolated in a single frequency. Mon´o´chro´mat´ic means, literally, one colour or the production of a single electromagnetic wavelength.

Light has a whole new application within the medical field. Although the FDA has not approved many of its potential uses, and current approvals are very limited, Europeans and Japanese have not been shy to push forward in this new science. There has been overwhelming success treating brain tumours, esophageal and lung cancers using photodynamic therapy.

When a light frequency is separated into a single wavelength it has profound dynamics. One of these known dynamics is its ability to travel vast distances within a single concentrated beam we know as the laser. It is said that in the mid-1970's Russians were the first to analyze cellular change to tissue using monochromatic light. A single light wave is essential, because cell tissue will not respond if more than one wavelength is present.

Dr. Robert Temple of the FDA has stated that patients with large tumours are left with no other options. PDT (photodynamic therapy) or LLLT (low level light therapy) relieves not only the symptoms but cures the problem. The process is so cost effective and efficient that it may have a negative impact on the pharmaceutical industry in the near future. Scientists have determined that photon energy is absorbed by the DNA, activating it. The DNA then transmits this new energy to the cell walls by means of protein and calcium transfer. Then the cell walls transform themselves into healthy shapes allowing the cell to function again at full capacity. The irradiated tissue increases blood flow helping to carry vitamins and nutrients into the areas where (they are) needed most, with no damage to surrounding tissue. As a result of the increased blood flow toxins and metabolic by-products are taken away from the suffering tissue quickly, thus stimulating damaged and irregular cell tissue into an accelerated healing process.

The single waveform light can perform near miracles in curing cancer, disintegrating tumours and repairing damaged tissue. This process can be done without painful surgery. The only known side effect to light therapy is a tendency for patients to sunburn easily, which can be avoided by staying out of direct sunlight for a 4 to 6 weeks after treatment.

NASA uses this technology on their space missions, and the Navy also uses monochromatic light with their special forces and on submarines. In space even a small nick won't heal. Prolonged weightlessness reduces the body' ability to repair itself, which leads to health risks in space.

There are several biotechnology companies now developing not only devices but photo-active chemicals knows as photosensitizers; photoreactive drugs that assist the light in its healing process. Bowling Green State University in Ohio has recently developed a Ph.D. program in the photochemical sciences. Most biostimulation devices have not yet been approved by the FDA. It is illegal for manufacturers in the U.S. to make claims of any clinical effectiveness.

Monochromatic light therapy has been used successfully in treatment of throat cancer, skin, lung and esophageal cancer. It is also good for pain relief, reduced swelling, sports injuries, macular degeneration, tendinitis, burns, herpes, among many other things.

Chapter 11

Controversy on Living on Light

Here are various reports on the deaths resulting from the practice of Living on Light and Jasmuheen's response to the deaths.

Guru's 'Air' Diet Proves Hard to Stomach
The Times (London), April 6, 2000 by Gillian Harris

A New Age guru who claims to have survived for seven years on herbal tea and chocolate digestive biscuits received a hostile reception last night when she delivered a lecture about her cult, which advocates continuous fasting. Jasmuheen, an Australian whose real name is Ellen Greve, arrived at Edinburgh University to talk to students about "breatharianism" whose followers live on "liquid light" and 300 calories a day.

It was her first visit to Britain since the death of Verity Linn, 49, whose emaciated body was found by the shores of Loch Cam, Sutherland, last September.

Ms Linn starved to death after embarking on a 21-day fast which was part of her induction into the cult. Opponents of Jasmuheen gathered outside the university's Chaplaincy Centre to accuse the cult leader of promoting eating disorders among vulnerable young people. They included Robin Harper, a Green MSP and rector of the university, who said: "I believe that one person and perhaps more have already been unwise enough to try some of this woman's ideas and died as a result."

However, Jasmuheen, a mother of two, said on Scot FM that she felt no responsibility for any of the four deaths around the world which have been linked to her teachings.

She said that Verity Linn, died of "exhaustion and exposure" which had nothing to do with her fast. During the lecture, Jasmuheen told her audience that she last ate a proper meal in 1993 and claimed that she survived by "tapping into an alternative source of nourishment" which came from within.

She denied that she was exposed as a fraud on an Australian television programme which revealed that she fell ill when she was filmed continuously without food.

"I flatly deny that I was ill," she said.

Breatharianism, which is practised by Tibetan monks but for shorter periods, has about 5,000 adherents worldwide. They believe that the elements contained in air—nitrogen, carbon dioxide, oxygen and hydrogen—can sustain a body. However, Jasmuheen, a former computer programmer, gave warning that it takes years of practice. On GMTV, Dr. Hilary Jones attacked her teachings. "When we have an epidemic of eating disorders in the Western world, you saying you can live off divine light and less than 300 calories a day is frankly dangerous." Although Jasmuheen claims that she has no trouble living without food, some of her followers find it more difficult. Two years ago one of her disciples in Australia was photographed coming out of a fast food shop munching on a chicken pie.

And an Australian journalist who was checking on to a flight with Jasmuheen was surprised to hear the airline attendant ask the cult leader to confirm that she had ordered a vegetarian meal. Jasmuheen quickly denied it, then changed her mind. "Yes, I did but I won't be eating it," she said.

We New Age Gurus have Got to Eat, at least Some of us do

The Express, September 25, 1999

Baffled by Feng shui? Undernourished by Breatharianism? Then let me lead you through to New Age enlightenment, David Robson at large as a spiritual guide advising those hungry for wisdom.

Are you sitting comfortably? In a chair that is kind to your spine? or are you in the lotus position perhaps? The room you are in—good feng shui? The colours—are they friendly? And have you breakfasted? On organic muesli? And herbal tea? Are you as relaxed as you might be? Have you soothed yourself with essential oils? Are the planets favourable? Your biorhythms in harmony? Yes, I believe they are. I can feel the positive vibrations from here. You are certainly approaching the state where reading this will become rewarding. But not too fast now! Always remember that your time is your own, a blessed possession.

Time is eternal, clocks are merely digital.

Before you begin to read my words, please join me in today's meditation from Conversations With God by my fellow spreader of enlightenment, Neale Donald Walsch, sage of Oregon (1.5 million copies sold worldwide): "See the Divine in a baby who needs changing at 3 am...in a bill that needs paying by the first of the month. Recognise the hand of God in the job that's lost..." Perhaps now you are in a state to imbibe my sentences, savour their goodness, feel their power, experience their essential grace. And if their wisdom is not apparent to you, remember this—you are but one tiny grain among millions, for my readers are as numerous as the sands of the desert and my words informed by the souls of generations of masters. The elevation of my mind and refinement of my thought are, in one sense, merely the fruit of many years of study; in another, they are the legacy of countless centuries. For who can guess what I was in former lives?

So come. My ability to guide you is to me a source of delight. Nothing, except my humility, gives me more pride. For only the poor of spirit cannot see the wisdom of my words. And if my paragraphs provoke bad feelings, remember this: it must be something within you, negativity blinding you to the light.

We will work together to open your mind. It may not happen immediately. We may need a new diet and a good deal of laying on of hands; with your goodwill we shall get there. But first open your purse: the willingness to hand over money is very often the prelude to enlightenment. You probably think this is easy—dispensing wisdom in what's known as the New Age. When the Prime Minister's wife wears a crystal and political pollsters keep The Road Less Travelled at their bedside, when every fashion designer's a Buddhist and Tesco has gone organic; when a total eclipse and the millennium come within months of each other, when the Government puts domes before homes. What more, you say, could a guru ask for? When Madonna studies the ancient wisdom of Kabalah, when neither homosexuality nor homeopathy raises an eyebrow, when The Little Book of Calm has replaced Wicked Willy as loo reading, is this not the open door? I understand. I always understand. But you too must understand. Untoward things happen. An Australian woman who had gone to Scotland to live in the spiritual community of Findhorn was found dead last week. Her efforts at Breatharian "self-cleansing" had led to starvation. She was discovered on a remote hillside with a diary logging her 21-day fast and telling how, even as she set out on a climbing and camping expedition, she felt weak for lack of food and water.

This is not, as they were quick to say, the Findhorn way. In fact, among the signs of the community's rude health is near-celestial success with organic vegetables. "Visitors often comment on how good our food is," said the Foundation's manager, distancing himself from the fatality. "This is the first we have heard of Breatharianism." An isolated incident it may have been, but it made for a rocky week on the road to Nirvana.

On Wednesday evening the former Ellen Greve of Brisbane, now Jasmuheen, mother of Breatharianism, author of *Living on Light, The Source of Nourishment For The New Millennium,* was on Newsnight, interviewed by Jeremy Paxman (the beneficiary of assertiveness training, unless I am much mistaken). There is no need for food, says Jasmuheen, you can draw your strength from chi-energy. (When, as she writes in her book, your four bodies—the physical, emotional, mental and spiritual—are in tune.) "This is nonsense," snapped Paxman. "If you don't eat, you die." The 21-day fast, which is the prelude to giving up food completely, is not something to rush into. It is the end of a progress through a vegetarian, then a raw food, then a wholly liquid diet. Jasmuheen prepared herself for years.

A few words about her book, just in case you happen not to have it. It is full of the language of ancient wisdom: her guidance came from the Ascended Masters, who have assured her that the body needs only Liquid Light. At the time of her writing she was still socialising over cups of tea. "When I am able to stop drinking without feeling that I am denying myself, I will do so, for I wish to take every step of the way in joy, with ease and grace."

She also says, at the beginning of Chapter Six: "It is interesting to note that ageing and death can still be experienced by breatharians." I suppose that "interesting" is perhaps not the word that Mr. Paxman, or indeed you, beloved reader, would choose, though wisdom tells us that death may be the most interesting experience of all.

Jasmuheen's words do not go unread. At Watkins Books—"specialists in mysticism, occultism, oriental religions, astrology, perennial wisdom, contemporary spirituality and Jungian psychology" off Charing Cross Road in the West End of London—they sell about 20 copies a month. Some time ago, Jasmuheen visited the shop. There were those on the staff who were sceptical about her. "I haven't taken nourishment from food for the last three years," she said. But is that the same as saying she had not eaten they wondered. This sort of thing, brothers and sisters in light, makes for bad karma. And the day-to-day travails of making a living purveying wisdom and healing are challenging enough without it. We gurus have got to eat too, you know (most of us anyway). And what a load we have to bear these days. I remember the time, in the Sixties when young hippies and eccentric old ladies were the only ones who needed us. How, in a blink of the eternal eye, things have changed! We have become society's emergency service, bringing help where all else fails.

Above the ruins of British society we float, above the wreckage of the old health service, the empty Christian churches, the schools where education has died, the offices where people lose themselves in work and the clubs where they lose themselves in idleness, the stores where they look for salvation through shopping and the bedrooms where they struggle for salvation through sex. All we see are unhappy faces. Western science with its bogus claims of all-knowingness has left people feeling empty and lost; conventional doctors, who cannot see beyond the symptoms of illness, and were long ago shorn of any aura of loving care, leave people feeling unhealed; teachers and priests, trapped in the deathly grip of

Christian dualism, detaching the body from the spirit, offer only benighted delusion. Now there is an acupuncturist on every corner; and a harvest of biofeedback, biogenics and cranial osteopathy. The business is there all right, but allow me in all humility to share something with you. Sometimes such is the loss of faith in the ways of the West that we Understanding Ones are faced with challenges even we do not understand. Let me tell you a story: a young family found that the light bulbs in their house were burning out with unwonted regularity.

Spiritually enlightened people who would never think of consulting the worldly ones at the electricity board, they called upon a practitioner of feng shui. Was it a challenge too far? Only time will tell. But when they came to me with their question I offered them only the honesty of my wisdom.

"How many feng shui practitioners does it take to change a light bulb?" they asked. My answer was: "It depends if the lightbulb wants to change." And oh, though life is eternal, it is forever changing. And while the spirit is everywhere, it doesn't help much with your business plan. For how is a guru to thrive in the spiritual supermarket with 100 varieties to choose from, where last year's paganism is this year's shamanism, where graphology all too soon gives way to iridology as a window to the soul? At this precise moment there is an abundance of angels in the ascendant who, we are told, can take away all our ills and are said to be very good with cars. The life of Dr. Doreen Virtue, author of *Angel Therapy*, changed when angels miraculously intervened and saved her from a car-jacking; Joan Wester Anderson, author of *Where Angels Walk*, became an angel-lover when angels rescued her son from a broken-down car in a blizzard without leaving tracks.

For those thereabouts, incidentally, next Tuesday is

Angel Day at The Tabernacle, Powys Square, London W11 (35 for a six-hour workshop). I could go into angels myself I suppose but will I be too late? It is all too likely they will have flown.

And so dear reader, this is indeed the age of abundance in the Guidance and Feeling market and, provided that you do nothing that bankrupts you or permanently damages your health, you may well find something that makes your life feel more harmonious—be it learning methods of contemplation, levitation or tofu cooking. As for me, I am very wise and very weary. I yearn for the simple days of yore when my only devotees were drugged-out hippies, when you had to go to health food shops to find brown rice, when GM meant General Motors. And my only pleasure was tantric sex.

I Haven't Eaten for 5 Years
Electronic Telegraph, October 24, 1999

Doctors and dieticians dismiss her claims as dangerous gobbledegook and a woman has died trying to convert to her breatharian creed. But Jasmuheen still insists that she 'lives on light'. Barbie Dutter meets her.

JASMUHEEN dances to the door in a leopard-print sundress that showcases an outstanding figure for a 41-year-old. She is curvaceous, with a slender waist and peachy complexion. Her eyes are bright, her hair glossy, her teeth white and strong. And she claims not to have eaten for five years.

We sit on the veranda of her Brisbane home, overlooking a generous pool, and sip blackcurrant and vanilla tea. This is her one concession to ingestion—two cups of tea a day, and the occasional glass of water. Or so she says.

She remembers quite clearly the last nutritious morsel to pass her lips—a lightly toasted, perfectly spiced felafel from a Lebanese health food shop. Then, she insists, she stopped eating forever.

Jasmuheen is a breatharian, the public face of a strange phenomenon called "living on light". She claims she tuned her body in 1993 to be spiritually receptive to an alternative, intangible form of nourishment called prana, or liquid light. On this basis, she says, she does not need to eat, never feels hungry and has gone without any food—with the exception of the odd chocolate biscuit to satisfy a stubborn taste-craving—for more than five years.

If this seems an outlandish assertion, there are even more fantastic claims to come. That this "pranic nourishment" could be the solution to global famine.

That it parallels the discovery that the Earth is round. That Jasmuheen is a messenger of the Ascended Masters, with whom she communicates through cosmic telepathy and who instructed her to attract public attention through the media to the cause of world hunger.

Her home, with its sunshine-yellow walls and pungent scent of incense, overflows with ancient and new-age icons. A gallery of "the Ascended Ones"—Christ, Krishna, Babaji, St. Germain, the Dalai Lama and more—adorns the walls. Their presence seems awkward alongside the material trappings of a fully equipped gym, sauna and dance room. But Jasmuheen attributes her glowing health not only to the lack of toxicity in her body, but to a daily routine of meditation and exercise involving hour upon hour of workouts, weight-training and aerobics.

All this on no food? Nonsense, declare the nutritionists. Physically impossible, proclaim the doctors. Morally irresponsible, cry the dieticians, concerned that she is preaching a message that will encourage dangerous weight loss or give anorexics their much-coveted excuse not to eat.

Jasmuheen's answer to such medical scepticism is this: "If a doctor told me it was physically impossible to survive without eating, I would say: 'Yes, according to your research it is. But not according to mine'."

So the research on which the health-care profession relies is flawed? "No, it is 100 percent correct. However, it does not take into account the fact that there are alternative forms of nourishment."

But, as a physical being, how is it possible to live without physical forms of nutrition?

"I do have nutrition—but from another source. If you put another nourishment source into your body, or release another nourishment source from within your body, then you don't need vitamins, minerals, nutrition from food.

"The point here is what form of nourishment you are taking. When you tune yourself—through meditation, through physical exercise, through dietary choices—then the signals that you are transmitting, as a bio-energetic system, are altered. The ability to live on light comes as a direct result of tuning those signals."

She claims the Christian definition of pranic nourishment would be that a person is "fed by the light of God". What would an atheist say? "That you have boosted the voltage of electro-magnetic energy in the body." Bamboozled, I ask to examine the contents of her fridge. She flings open the door with a flourish and an array of shiny, healthy food confronts us—brown bread and beansprouts, pawpaw and hummus, half a dozen cartons of soya milk and jar upon jar of cooking sauces. "It's Jeff's food," she announces. Jeff is her fiancè, a vegan, who cooks and eats. A quick glance around the kitchen reveals a well-used chopping board, a shelf jostling with herbs and condiments and—aha!—a dozen bottles of vitamins and supplements. "They're Jeff's. I don't need vitamins. I get all the vitamins I need."

Jasmuheen is a new-ager who is relatively unknown in her native Australia but hugely successful in Germany.

She has written eight books on self-empowerment, mind-mastery and, more recently, living on light, but claims to make little money from her work, re-investing any royalties into spreading the word. Her home in the smart, hillside suburb of Chapel Hill was, however, purchased through the proceeds of her books.

Next month she will bring her message to Britain, and is confident her work will be embraced worldwide. She has even been tipped off—by an angelic source—that she will be invited on The Oprah Winfrey Show. She claims her spiritual mentor, St. Germain, told her to use the fact of not needing to eat to harness media attention. "He's my etheric Press officer," she says, giggling at my look of earthly incomprehension.

She is unswerving in her claim that her life is food-free. She is also somewhat smug in the knowledge that these claims are impossible to prove-short of being locked in a laboratory or having a minder with her every second of every day.

As we talk, there is a rustle of plastic in the kitchen, signalling Jeff's arrival home with some groceries. Jasmuheen seizes the moment delightedly to remind me that her life is free of such mundane chores.

"I have no shopping, I have no cooking, I have no cleaning, I have no dishes. I have endless extra time because I don't have to worry about food. When you're not eating you don't need to sleep much, so I have 20 hours a day to play with. It's wonderful."

Jasmuheen was born Ellen Greve in the Snowy Mountains of New South Wales, the fifth and youngest child of Norwegian migrants who came to Australia after the Second World War. She dropped out of an art degree after less than a year, and became pregnant at 19 while waitressing in Sydney to save money "to do the hippy trail".

She married the father of her baby (the first of two daughters who are now apparently supportive of their mother's mission) but the marriage foundered after seven years and she took a job in the finance industry, earning a salary substantial enough to pay for a nanny, private schooling for her daughters and an Alfa Romeo.

In 1992, she lost her job, and began to focus on her interest in meditation and mind-mastery. She held workshops and seminars, began writing and sold her home and car to make ends meet. It was around this time, during a meditation session, that a message "came through" to stop eating food. Already a vegetarian of two decades, she prepared herself by refining and reducing her intake until all she was eating was a little soup. She then put herself through a punishing 21-day conversion course with no food or fluids for the first seven days and occasional sips of orange juice and water for the remaining 14. This course, which she co-pioneered and writes about extensively in her latest book *Living on Light*, attracted controversy in July when an Australian woman, attempting to convert to Breatharianism, collapsed and died in hospital 10 days later. The dead woman's tutor—a 60-year-old Brisbane man whom Jasmuheen claims never to have met but is referred to in her book—is awaiting trial for unlawful killing.

Jasmuheen admits the course is dangerous, and insists it is only for "spiritual warriors" who have prepared themselves through years of meditation and exercise, who have weaned themselves off their emotional dependency on food and have a basic grasp of quantum physics. She rejects accusations of moral irresponsibility, saying she has publicly warned those with weight problems or anorexia against the process. She says that they could not complete the conversion anyway. "If people are not coming from a place of integrity and the right motivation then it doesn't work."

Dr. Sandra Capra, a senior lecturer at the School of Public Health at the Queensland University of Technology and President of the Dieticians Association of Australia, describes Jasmuheen's claims as meaningless mumbo-jumbo. "It's like me saying the moon is a rocky substance that orbits the Earth, and somebody else saying the moon is made of cheese. It would be impossible for her to still be alive on what she claims her intake to be. You don't have to eat—you can survive on a well-planned liquid diet—but you cannot survive without nutrients. I think this message is appalling because it misleads people and it is dangerous."

Dr. Capra says total abstinence from food and fluids is considered highly dangerous after three to four days. The maximum accepted time for a person to survive with no fluids is six days. In a period of weeks, with no nutrients, repercussions could include symptoms of scurvy and beri beri; changes in the blood leading to headaches, dizziness and the increased threat of strokes; disturbance to the cardio-vascular system, increasing the risk of heart attacks; major metabolic problems, brain disorders and coma.

"This individual claims there are about 5,000 breatharians internationally, but cannot name any. She says there have been studies, but cannot name any. I can't tell if she's a true believer or a liar, but this is gobbledegook."

The only way for Jasmuheen to quieten her critics would be to submit to clinical tests, she says. Jasmuheen responds that in August 1999, during a 33-day retreat— yet to be arranged—in Germany or France, she and about 30 other breatharians will submit to the full scrutiny of medical professionals, scientists and the media. But she says she will not have tests beforehand because the results would be dismissed as a "one-off miracle".

As the founder and mouthpiece of a number of

Internet-based outfits—the Self Empowerment Academy, the Cosmic Internet Academy, the Movement of an Awakened Positive Society—Jasmuheen is beefing up her international profile with lecture tours, such as the one in London in late November.

She is scholarly in metaphysics and Eastern philosophy and articulate in her arguments. Her analogies are a peculiar mixture of the esoteric and the technical. "The body has cellular memory like computer software. If you change what you want to achieve, you've got to change the program. So if people have a program that says: 'If I don't eat or drink I'll die or waste away to nothing', then they'll die or waste away to nothing. But you can reprogram the body by changing your belief systems."

She says that she has suffered little weight loss—around 9 lb—because of such a reprogramming process. "I decided that when my weight dropped below 47 kilos I looked like a Biafran, so I commanded the body to stabilize at a minimum of 47 kilos and it did."

She says her social life has suffered from the lack of invitations to dinner parties. She regrets her fiance's frustration in not being able to express his love by cooking. I wonder if she conducts midnight raids on Jeff's goodies, or keeps muesli bars stashed under her mattress. I ask if she has bowel movements.

She is unfazed. "It may be rabbit-type droppings every three weeks if I am just drinking, or a little more if I nibble once a week. There is little to eliminate, except for dead cells and pollutants."

On this note I leave—and head for the nearest McDonald's.

Face behind Food-Free Teaching
Jasmuheen's book about living on "God's light" *The London Times*, September 21, 1999 by Susie Steiner

Jasmuheen, 42, a blonde Brisbane spiritualist,

teaches that nourishment can come from light, and that this can help to solve world famine. "I have found another form of nourishment. It's called Pranic light, which is the light of God found all over the Universe and inside everyone," she says.

Jasmuheen believes she is a messenger of the Ascended Masters, with whom she communicates through cosmic energy. The guru is said to have converted more than 5,000 people to her foodless diet. Most live in Germany.

She is expanding her empire in Britain. Her book, *Living on Light,* is published here next month, and she is conducting a lecture tour in November. Jasmuheen also has a website called the Cosmic Internet Academy.

On it she writes: Every second second a child dies from hunger-related disease. This is unnecessary and a group of dedicated, tough, well-trained, self-selected warriors (known also as the Knights of Camelot)_have been utilising themselves as guinea pigs to prove that human beings do not need food to live."

She admits drinking water, fruit juice and tea, and nibbles on a chocolate biscuit a few times a year. Eating, she says, is permissible for pleasure, as long as it is not out of need.

She accepts that giving up food is a delicate process and believes in a strict 21-day conversion.

Yesterday her spokesman, Gerd Lange, said Jasmuheen could not be held responsible for the death in Scotland, because the victim cannot have followed the 21-day process guidelines properly.

"It is not for Joe Bloggs who has a hamburger down the pub. It's for people who have a spiritual interest."

Movement whose Followers 'Live on Light'
Newswire, September 21, 1999

Breatharianism is a relatively new and little-known movement founded by an Australian woman called Ellen Greve.

It is based on the concept of "breatharianism", which promotes the idea of living on light and almost entirely without food and liquids. Followers are encouraged not to try the process without spiritual, emotional and physical training, as unless they have the right motivation they will fail.

When people first decide they want to adopt this way of living, they are encouraged to cut down slowly on their food and liquid intake before undergoing what Jasmuheen terms the "21-day programme" of spiritual cleansing during which they eat and drink practically nothing.

Mrs. Greve, who lives in Brisbane and is married with two daughters, claims to have been living on herbal tea, juice and the occasional biscuit since 1993 after being told to change her life by her spiritual mentor, St Germain.

Mrs. Greve changed her name to Jasmuheen as her devotion to the way of living developed. She has produced a range of materials, including books and videos, to spread her ideas and claims around 5,000 followers worldwide.

Despite the fact she is relatively unknown, when she came to London last year to promote her latest book, called *Living on Light*, around 400 people turned up to hear one of her speeches.

Michelle Shirley, administrator of the Cult Information Centre, said the movement could not be legitimately described as a cult as people were not coerced into joining against their own will through techniques such as brainwashing.

She said Jasmuheen spread her philosophy through books, speaking tours, videos and the Internet, and it was down to individuals themselves to decide if they wanted to adopt her teachings.

The movement attracted controversy in Australia

following the death of a woman who attempted to adopt its teachings.

Ms. Shirley said she was extremely concerned about the possible spread of the movement in the UK.

Fresh-Air Dietician Fails TV Show's Challenge
Yahoo News, October 25, 1999

A Dietician who claims it is possible to live off fresh air has failed in a television documentary to practise what she preaches.

An Australian programme, 60 Minutes, asked Jasmuheen, a former financial adviser whose real name is Ellen Greve, to demonstrate that she could live healthily without any nutrients other than air for one week.

Last month, Verity Linn, an Australian environmentalist, was found starved to death by a loch in West Sutherland with a copy of the teachings of Jasmuheen in her belongings. Ms. Linn died one week after beginning a planned three-week fast.

Jasmuheen, who claims not to have eaten real food for years, agreed to be cut off from the outside world for the test. But the programme-makers were forced to call a halt to the trial after four days when she showed signs of becoming seriously ill.

Jasmuheen had initially been confined to a hotel room in Brisbane with teams of female security guards in constant attendance. Her progress was checked by a female doctor, Dr. Berris Wink, president of the Queensland branch of the Australian Medical Association.

But when she began showing signs of stress, high blood pressure and dehydration after just 48 hours, the self-styled guru blamed it not on food and fluid deprivation, but polluted air.

The cult leader claimed that her confinement close to a busy main road meant she could not get the nutrients she needed to survive as a Breatharian. Dr. Wink told her she was already clearly suffering the effects of dehydration. "You are now over 5 per cent dehydrated. If we let this go much longer, that's going to damage your kidney," she said. 60 Minutes moved Jasmuheen on day three to a mountainside retreat about 15 miles away from the city , where she was filmed enjoying the fresh air she said she could now live on happily. However, as the filming progressed, it became obvious that Jasmuheen was becoming ill. Her speech was slow, her pupils dilated and she had lost almost a stone. One doctor advising 60 Minutes urged Jasmuheen and the programme to stop the challenge. After four days, Jasmuheen told the programme's presenter, Richard Carlton: "I feel really good, now I'm here. Well, I look like I've lost a lot of weight and the doctor confirms that." Dr. Wink told her: "You are now quite dehydrated, probably over 10 percent, getting up to 11 percent." She also announced: "Her pulse is about double what it was when she started. The risks if she goes any further are kidney failure. 60 Minutes would be culpable if they encouraged her to continue. She should stop now."

Jasmuheen challenged the decision, saying: "Look, 6,000 people have done this around the world without any problem." She blamed 60 Minutes for putting her beside a busy main road at the start of the experiment. "I asked for fresh air. Seventy per cent of my nutrients come from fresh air. I couldn't even breath," she said.

Dr. Wink told the programme, which decided not continue the test after the four-day period: "Unfortunately there are a few people who may believe what she says, and I'm sure its only a few, but I think it's quite irresponsible for somebody to be trying to encourage others to do something that is so detrimental to their health."

Next month an Australian doctor and his wife who

say they are Breatharians are due to go on trial charged with manslaughter after a woman died in their care.

All They Need is the Air...
BBC News, September 22, 1999

Members of a little-known cult claim that all they need is the air that they breathe. Breatharians claim to be nourished by prana, a Hindu term for the universal life force.

Their leader Jasmuheen, a 42-year-old New Age guru from Brisbane formerly known as Ellen Greve, says she has eaten little more than herbal tea, juice and an occasional biscuit since 1993. She instead draws energy from prana and meditation.

Yet the cult has been implicated in at least two deaths. The most recent, Australian-born Verity Linn, 49, was found dead in a remote part of the Scottish Highlands on 16 September.

Police believe she was following the Breatharians' 21-day fast. A diary belonging to Ms. Linn recorded her last days as she refused to eat or drink, believing it would "spiritually cleanse" her body and "recharge her both physically and mentally".

Another woman died in an Australian hospital after following the Breatharian 21-day fast.

Pure Energy
Breatharianism relies on light and taking in only tiny amounts of food and liquid.

Followers believe that the energy they save on metabolising food and fluid can be redirected into physical, emotional and spiritual energy. "We are neither a religion nor a cult, just concerned citizens who have experienced from our association with the Ascended Masters, and many other great Ones and teachers," Jasmuheen says on her website. "Our work is to share some cosmic, yet intelligent alternatives that offer pragmatic solutions to many of the challenges that face the world today."

She claims to have hit upon a solution to world hunger —that in time, we can all learn to live on air alone.

The Breatharians' findings—based on surveys of those who have completed the 21-day fast and interviews with alternative health practitioners-will be published in late 1999.

Jasmuheen plans to send the finished report to agencies such as the United Nations and UNICEF, "to provide a step-by-step programme to eliminate world hunger, improve global health and well being, [and] decrease pollution".

She hopes to overturn the "outdated" view of the majority of the world's population that 'if you don't eat, you must die'. Spread the word Many of the Breatharians' ideas are based on the teachings of St. Germain, a 16th century European monk and alchemist, through his writings and "more recent channelled material".

His profile on the website is quite a read: "Many would know of St. Germain as the writer of William Shakespeare's plays. Previous embodiments are said to include Merlin and Christopher Columbus". The learned saint himself encouraged Jasmuheen to promote Breatharianism, using modern-day technology and media contacts to spread the word world-wide.

'Not Strictly a Cult'

Michelle Shirley, spokeswoman for the Cult Information Centre, says that although Breatharianism is not strictly a cult, the centre has been monitoring its activities.

"A cult uses coercive teaching. We don't have any evidence that that is being used here, or that it isn't being used.

"Jasmuheen is a spiritual teacher who spreads her words through the Internet and her books. So it is not an organisation that you join, it is more fluid than that."

Friends and families of Breatharians have contacted the centre five times in the past year.

They are encouraged to be as non-confrontational as possible, as Jasmuheen's followers are told that they should not be swayed by negative comments.

"We are particularly concerned about any implication that if it doesn't work, it is the person's fault," Ms. Shirley says. "That implies there is nothing wrong with the Breatharians' teachings."

Jasmuheen's Response

Germany, July 1999, from the Author of the controversial book *"Living on Light"*, Jasmuheen, issued by the Self Empowerment Academy, P.O. Box 737, Kenmore 4069 Australia.

"Goodness is the only investment that never fails." Henry David Thoreau—US Author and naturalist

Hi! I am writing to you all in response to the recent controversy about my book *"Living on Light"* among certain media in Germany. *"Focus"* magazine is concerned about the death of a man in Germany that occurred some 3 months before my book was published. This is exactly why I wrote the book in the first place.

Insufficient information on the initiation that I then outline further in the book, had begun to be circulated globally and I felt that this could have detrimental effects. As many know, it's hard to control the release of information that just wants to get out there because this is what freedom of speech is all about. Yet we can make sure that information is released responsibly.

We also need to make sure that our research sources

are confirmed to be from a credible source. *"Focus"* magazine has not bothered to check their facts and will no doubt make their apologies for this shortly to their readers. This is not the first time this has happened with German media. A leading new age magazine also neglected to investigate whether the information they printed on our work 6 months ago was true or just unsubstantiated rumour. Unfortunately for their readers it was just rumor. While this lack of ethics surprised me considering their business focus, we chose to ignore this but will not ignore it again.

So let us look at some facts. Many individuals are attracted to the idea of being free from the need to eat food. Others desire to be free from all external attachments and seeking enlightenment, begin to make adjustments to their lifestyles. In M.A.P.S. we call these people the Ambassadors of Light and yes I am one. M.A.P.S. is the movement of people who are committed to finding positive solutions to many modern day challenges. After over 20 years of metaphysical study, I accidentally discovered prana as an alternative source of nourishment. I have discovered since through 6 years of personal in-depth research, that the lifestyle we live that frees us from the need for food, could have very positive applications to world health and world hunger challenges.

We are not promoting the 21-day process to society, we are promoting the power of the Divine One Within us all. By its Grace only can we be fed like this. We are not saying that stopping to eat food will end world hunger and world health problems. We are saying that the lifestyle that allows us to now to be able to live on light, will do this. All this is covered in my final book on this field of research *"Ambassadors of Light—Living on Light"* that KOHA Verlag will publish in the next few months. In this book we advocate the benefits of vegetarianism particularly for its health benefits, and its long term global resource sustainability benefits. We look in depth at the redistribution of our resources—at disarmament, pharmaceutical use and prohibition laws. We provide research from the Qigong Masters on their ability to live without food and we provide other medical research that has been conducted on this since the 1920's.

Yes we promote vegetarianism as one part of a lifestyle recipe that we suggest people adopt if they are interested in eventually living free from the need of food. We also promote it as part of our interest in the cessation of slaughter of all life on the planet. Our desire to connect with the Divine One Within allows a process of metamorphosis to begin in our lives, that we can control the speed of. We control the speed of change through diet, meditation and through physical, emotional, mental and spiritual exercise.

Mental exercise involves programming and mind mastery. Emotional exercise occurs through the way we co-exist in our relationships with each other. Spiritual exercise is the path all initiates take when they want to experience the 'enlightening' qualities of their DOW.

As we have often stated, the 21-day process is a placebo for living on light. It is instead a powerful spiritual initiation that is not to be taken lightly. This initiation, if prepared for well, can leave you in a state of grace and wonder at the majesty of life—its sole purpose is to connect you consciously on a much deeper level with your DOW. We trust you will enjoy our new book and ask for your support till then. Remember anyone prepared to challenge the status quo comes under scrutiny from time to time and also that the spreading of incorrect information is harmful to us all.

With love light and laughter—Jasmuheen Circulated by KOHA Verlag at the request of the Self Empowerment Academy, July 1999.

CHAPTER 12

Dancing with My DOW

In response to concerns over some individuals that have died during the 21-day process, Jasmuheen distributed an excerpt from her book *"Dancing with My DOW"*.

Below is an excerpt from my book *"Dancing with My DOW"* that explains what I know about these deaths.—Jas.

The woman who died in Australia—Lani Morris—did so while staying with a man and his wife who were subsequently arrested and charged with negligence. He is still awaiting trial and it will be up to the jury to decide if he was indeed in anyway responsible for her death and if he lacked the ability to discern that she was in need of medical care earlier than it was provided. Interviews with Mr. Pesnak and his wife share how Lani refused all of his help and attention for a number of days and he was loath to interfere with her free will and decision to continue. Her choice to go through the 21-day process is not the issue for the courts, the concern is that the 'caregiver' did not act soon enough to seek medical care for her. I have been working with the prosecution as an independent expert witness. I had never met nor been involved in any way with either the Pesnaks or Lani Morris. Immediately after this occurred the Self Empowerment Academy issued very strong guidelines imploring people to act responsibly at all times.

The next issue is the death of a German man, Timo Degan which occurred prior to both the publication of my book and my arrival in Germany. Apparently he had decided to do the process after reading the 21-day guidelines called "Choosing God over Illusion" that someone else had written that was already circulating the global scene. One of the main reasons I was guided to write the book initially was to make sure that people received more information than what these few guidelines were providing so I incorporated these previous guidelines—with a few elaborations—into my book. This book is now in 8 languages and covers issues like mind mastery, meditation, programming and releasing limited belief systems needed to be addressed. He died after having an epileptic fit and hitting his head against a bed. Again I had never met Timo as he had heard about the 21-day process through other sources. In dealing with the lawyer for *Focus* magazine in response to their incorrect reporting I was told it was my 'thesis', my process and thus I was to blame. This again is absolutely incorrect and a full investigation into this matter will prove this. It is not my thesis—I am the one who is in the public eye determined to see that people act responsibly if they choose this path and reporting on our research into this phenomena.

Recently we have the case of Verity Linn, a very switched on and dedicated woman who did exactly what she wanted to do—or so I am told by friends who knew her well at Findhorn. Apparently, according to her diary, she began the 21-day program then traveled and walked long distances against strong weather conditions to pitch her tent on the moorland. This is 100% not recommended in the 21-day process where it is stated that on page 131 in *"Living on Light-Nutrition for the New Millenium"* "once you commence this process, you are not to leave your immediate environment". Verity chose to begin—then expend incredible energy—on her journey to find her 'spot' unfortunately it was too much for her system and she died of weather exposure and not starvation. I would assume that her system was weakened by not eating and not drinking then doing so much physical activity. Obviously, Verity thought she was fit enough to begin the process, and not only 'leave her immediate environment' but also do so much physical activity. Sadly choosing to ignore the guidelines and did not expect to have trouble—a woman choosing to do this alone on the moors for 21 days is a much stronger one that I am and I would never recommend that this initiation be done in this way. We always say 'once you begin, you conserve all your energy—rest, relax, read, meditate, be still. This brings me to the point that the caliber of people involved in this needs to be assessed. I call them the Ambassadors of Light and while they come from many different spiritual backgrounds, all believe themselves to be their own master and it is insulting to say that I am their guru or leader. If anything I am just the media spokesperson whose talk is based on years of personal experience and research as shared in my new book on this topic—"Ambassadors of Light—Living on Light".

Research on External Prana

Prana is a Sanskrit word meaning 'breath'. It was a central conception in early Hindu philosophy, and was held to be the principle of vitality, the universal life force. The Chinese word for prana is 'qi' or 'ch'i' which has the same meaning. Early Taoists philosophers and alchemists regarded prana as a vital force existing in the breath and bodily fluids, and they developed techniques to alter and control the movement of prana within the body. Their purpose was to achieve physical longevity and spiritual power.

Chinese philosophers hold that prana was transformed through the Yang (active) and Yin (passive) modes in the five elements; wood, metal, earth, water and fire, which in turn formed the basic constituents of the physical universe.

Prana is the life energy which keeps the body alive and healthy. There are three major sources of prana: solar prana, air prana and ground prana. Solar prana is prana from sunlight which invigorates the whole body and promotes good health, and is obtained by exposure to sunlight, and by drinking water that has been exposed to sunlight. Air prana is absorbed by the lungs through breathing and also absorbed directly by the energy centres referred to esoterically as chakras. More air prana can be absorbed by deep, slow, rhythmic breathing than by short, shallow breathing. It can also be absorbed through the pores of the skin by persons who have reached a certain level of esoteric sophistication.

Ground prana is absorbed through the soles of the feet. This is done automatically and unconsciously. Walking barefoot increases the amount of ground prana absorbed by the body. Water absorbs prana from sunlight, air and the ground with which it comes in contact. Plants and trees absorb prana from sunlight, air, water and the ground. Men and animals can obtain prana from sunlight, air, ground, water and food. Fresh food contains more prana than preserved food.

Prana can also be projected to another person for healing. Persons with a lot of excess prana tend to make other people around them feel better and healthier.

However, those who are depleted tend unconsciously to absorb prana from other people. In recent years substantial scientific testing has been done to establish the presence and nature of pranic emissions. However, the methodology of modern science stresses that the observer and the observed are separate and this is an essential feature of scientific observation. But traditional prana theory stresses that according to the most fundamental reasoning, the observed and the observer are in fact one, both consisting of prana, and are inseparable.

Therefore, the observer alters what is observed by observing it, which is what in fact occurs at the level of quantum physics. This makes the accurate measurement of prana by traditional scientific methods difficult. In the scientific investigations conducted by the Chinese which are now being published in book form in English, it is noted that the external prana emitted by a practitioner, carries different information from the prana of a non-practitioner. It is well known that all body parts, internal organs and tissues of the human body have a weak magnetic field. However, when a pranic practitioner enters into a state of pranic emission, the magnetic intensity of certain places of the body surface can be ten thousand to one million times stronger than that of internal organs. That is, ten thousand to one million times stronger than a pranic non-practitioner. Numerous scientific tests conducted by Chinese scientists have established the most remarkable properties of prana, e.g., prana has been proved to be able to penetrate walls and tens of metres of dense material. Consequently, neutrons, neutrinos, gamma rays and x-rays were considered, because they had these properties. However, on testing it was found that prana was not exclusively any of these emissions.

Pranic healing was considered for many years to be a kind of psychological treatment, and this point of view is still quite popular in the west. There are some reasons behind it. For instance co-operation, especially psychological co-operation from the patient, is important during treatment. However, scientific experiments have shown that liquid crystal molecules rotate under the influence of external prana, thereby demonstrating that external pranic healing is not just a psychological treatment. It has objective effects independent of any psychological dimension. Numerous cases of pranic healing of an extraordinary nature are reported by Chinese scientific experiments, probably the most dramatic being the healing of bone fractures, with the bones being x-rayed both before and after the pranic treatment, and demonstrating the bones having knitted and healed within hours .

All experiments regarding external pranic treatment have to be made with the external prana emitted by pranic masters, that is healers or teachers in the field. Prana emission consumes the prana master's vital energy, and is subject to their physical and mental conditions. As a result only similar, but not identical results can be obtained from different pranic emissions. This makes the normal scientific observation process difficult. Further, external pranic experiments often produce results that seem difficult to explain using modern scientific knowledge and demonstrate unusual phenomenon that are often beyond common sense.

The nature of the external prana has been studied in China for over ten years, involving almost all fields of modern physics such as infra-red radiation, ultra-violet radiation, electro-magnetic waves, micro waves, magnetic fields, neutrons, electron physics and so on. However, those who have participated in the experiments suggest that the properties of external prana are still far beyond what may have been studied. It is obvious that there are physical properties of external prana yet to be discovered due to the limitations of our current understanding of science and technology. It was demonstrated that experiments using prana emissions can be conducted at a distance of 2,000 km. from the emitter of the prana to the experiment. This is difficult for science to comprehend. However, prana does not seem to obey the normal scientific rules pertaining to proportionality. It can probably be best compared with a laser beam which can travel long distances and not lose much intensity in its travels.

The point seems to be that there is no evidence that external prana is a gravitational or electro-magnetic force, and therefore does not necessarily obey the scientific law of proportionality. The conclusion of many scientific experiments is that before external prana reaches the sample being tested it does not have a definite form or state such as infra-red radiation, gamma rays or neutrons, instead it only has the general characteristics of external prana, such as penetrating, targeting and bi-directionality. Only at the moment it reaches and touches the sample being tested does the external prana acquire the definite state corresponding to the conditions required to change this sample in a predetermined way. For example, external prana may act like ultra violet light, infra-red radiation or neutrons to affect the object. Scientists call this characteristic "target-adaptability" of external prana. The relationship between western science and pranic masters is strained, to put it mildly, because the level of pranic practice is higher than that of modern science.

A pranic master pays close attention to consciousness and to the effect of the consciousness of an object. The observer and the observed are connected. This is something that traditional science opposes. To give an example, it is generally believed that without food and water a human will die in a short period of time, but a Chinese girl in New York has been in a state of 'Bigu' since 21 October, 1987 when she attended a prana emitting lecture by a prana master. At that time she was aged 10. Bigu is a state in which a person maintains a normal life with little or no intake of food or water. After

10 months from the start of her Biju, the Chinese Military Academy of Medicine organised eight medical experts to conduct a month long investigation of her. They reached the conclusion that in spite of her extremely insufficient intake of calories and nutrition she had maintained her normal life and growth and the stability of internal physiological conditions. A light duty worker normally needs 2,200 calories each day, but her daily nutrition consumption was only 200 to 300 calories each day, and calculations showed that according to her daily activities, that she needed at least 1500 calories per day. These facts seriously challenged modern physiology.

Another scientific oddity is the paradox of being able to move solid objects through barriers. A simplistic explanation is that an object with one dimensional freedom can only move back and forth on a straight line. If there is an obstacle on the line, the object cannot pass it. The object with two-dimensional freedom however, can easily pass around it. For an object being only able to move in a two-dimensional plane it will be stopped when it is surrounded by a circling obstacle. But an object with three-dimensional freedom can easily get over this circling obstacle from above and move on. It is natural to deduce that an object with four-dimensional freedom will not be hindered by an obstacle in a three-dimensional space. Therefore, pills sealed in a bottle, where the pills have four-dimensional freedom, would not be impeded by the three-dimensional bottle. The three-dimensional pills enter into a fourth dimensional space the instant they receive external prana emitted by a prana master who has extraordinary functions.

A Chinese scientist from the Institute of Space Medical Engineering captured the whole process of pills escaping from a bottle using a high speed camera. He found one frame of film among several thousand frames showing half of a pill coming out of the side of the bottle and the following three frames showing the whole pill gradually dropping down. The observers suggested that the instant a pill receives the external prana emitted by the prana master, it enters into a state of virtual mass thereby passing through the bottle without resistance and afterwards turns back into its original real state—a pill. They, of course, have no explanation as to why the pill goes into a fourth dimensional space or virtual mass space, after receiving the external prana.

Regarding how external prana can cause healing and a Bigu state, it is suggested that the average person has about 14-15 billion brain cells, but usually uses only 4-5% and never more than 30% of these cells. Even though as people age, they have memory failure, 80-90% of their brain cells remain unused at the time of their death. It has been observed that after a person enters into a state of exposure to external prana the neutrons in the deep layers of the cerebrum also enter into an excited state. This affects the regions of the brain where consciousness is focused. As a result the bio-electric currents in these regions are likely to be further enhanced. In other words, pranic practice activates the unused 80-90% of the brain cells by strengthening the brain's bio-electric currents. On entering a pranic state the consumption of oxygen decreases while at the same time the lungs' ability to absorb oxygen increases. As well, the capacity of tissues in the whole body to store oxygen and the capacity of the lungs is enhanced. Consequently, pranic practice is much more effective than athletic training. A long distance runner has lungs with large capacities, but also consumes large amounts of oxygen, and as a result cannot stay under water for very long. However, some people are able to stay alive while being buried underground in a coffin for 6 to 7 days. It is difficult to explain this phenomenon according to the lung capacity and oxygen needs of an ordinary person. However, it is explainable from a pranic perspective. In a pranicaly enhanced state a practitioner does not need much oxygen. Pranic practices increase inhaling efficiency and expand the storage capacity of the lung tissues. It also decreases the consumption of oxygen. At certain stages of practice some pranic practitioners eat very little, or do not eat all. This is because they are capable of transforming energy and making full use of stored energy to keep themselves alive. A few do not even drink water, for water can be absorbed through the skin pores.

One may question how a person can live without food. First, the gastric and internal fluid of pranic practitioners contain many nutrients. Second, everyone has nutrients stored in the body, yet most people do not know how to transform and utilise them. Many days may pass without eating food, yet one can still be energised by absorbing self transformed high energy substances. It is not a question of eating, but rather of absorbing nutrients in a different manner. One can utilise the body's accumulated nutrition and transfer it to gastric and intestinal fluids for high quality nourishment. Pranic practitioners do not merely absorb nutrients through their mouth and nose. They can use many other ways to absorb energy substances for nourishment. Water, for example, does not have to enter only through the mouth. Light does not have enter only through the eyes. Pranic practitioners absorb high energy substances from the universe that are unavailable to others. In this manner one can eat less or not eat at all for a length of time and still maintain a high energy level. When the absorption of high energy substances is enhanced, one may go without food for a long period of time. Thus pranic practices are an ideal way to improve the digestive system of the body. Only the earliest of scientific research has been done to date on the amazing possibilities that pranic practices offer. However, the Chinese are the leaders in this field, and ten years of their research is now being translated into English books which will be very educational for western science. The sources of research were: *"The Encyclopedia Britannica, Miracles through Pranic Healing* by Master Choa Kok Sui , and *Scientific Qigong Exploration* by Lu Zuyin."

CHAPTER 13

The Divine Dance for Paradise

Jasmuheen's European Tour Speech—November 1999

Hello and welcome to this gathering and the Divine Dance for Paradise. How many of you have previously attended my lectures and seminars? To you I say thank you for your continuing love and support. As some of you may be aware, the last few months for me have been particularly challenging, as I have become a target for the media in their bid to spread misinformation about my work. As this has arisen purely from their lack of awareness of the facts and research already done in this field, it is easy to forgive them, for what some have not yet come to realize, is that paradise is in humanity's blueprint of evolution.

For me personally, this period of time has been an amazing journey that has required trust and strength, clarity of commitment, and also great courage, and yet to continue on in the face of so much adversity is nothing new for many. Galileo, Gandhi, Martin Luther King and thousands of others, known and unknown, have been challenging the status quo since there was a status quo to challenge. As the German philosopher, Arthur Schopenhauer said: "All truth passes through three stages. First, it is ridiculed. Second, it is violently opposed. Third, it is accepted as being self-evident."

Schopenhauer, like myself was a student of the Vedas, from which the very first information about prana has come. Prana is the energy behind the breath, it is also the energy that allows the divine to dance so evidently within the universe. Albert Einstein once said : The most beautiful thing we can experience is the mysterious. It is the source of true art and science. He to whom the emotion is stranger, who can no longer pause to wonder and stand wrapped in awe, is as good as dead; his eyes are closed. The insight into the mystery of life, coupled though it be with fear, has also given rise to religion. To know what is impenetrable to us really exists, manifesting itself as the highest wisdom and the most radiant beauty, which our dull faculties can comprehend only in their most primitive forms—this knowledge, this feeling is at the center of true religiousness. There is an old Vedic story about Prana that we find in various Upanishads. The five main faculties of our nature—the mind, breath (prana), speech, ear and eye—were arguing with each other as to which one of them was the best and most important. This reflects the ordinary human state in which our faculties are not integrated but fight with each other, competing for their rule over our attention. To resolve this dispute they decided that each would leave the body and see whose absence was most missed.

First speech left the body but the body continued though mute. Next the eye left but the body continued though blind. Next the ear left but the body continued though deaf. Mind left but the body continued though unconscious. Finally the Prana began to leave and the body began to die and all the other faculties began to lose their energy. So they all rushed to Prana and told it to stay, lauding its supremacy. Clearly Prana won the argument. Prana gives energy to all our faculties, without which they cannot function. Without honoring Prana first, there is nothing else we can do, and no energy with which to do anything. Some people call prana Qi, others call it God, as many of you are aware from reading my

writings, I call it the Divine One Within—our DOW. Yes
it is true that I am probably now known as one of the
more public researchers in the field of experiential study
of prana power. Other researchers are Choa Kok Sui,
head of the International Pranic Healers Association and
the Qi Master Dr. Yan Xin (Shin). I love Choa Kok Sui's
quote: An intelligent person is not closed minded.

He does not behave like an ostrich burying his head in
the ground trying to avoid new ideas and developments.
An intelligent person is not gullible. He does not accept
ideas blindly. He studies and digests them thoroughly,
then evaluates them against his reason; he tests these
new ideas and developments through experiments and
his experiences. An intelligent person studies these ideas
with a clear objective mind.

Choa Kok Sui's work, like Reiki, reveals the healing
power of prana. The work of Dr. Yan Xin when
understood, heralds a huge milestone for humanity at
this time. With over 60 books focused on the Qi Masters
research into the power of external Qi emissions, if all I
can do at this time is lead the world to his doorstep and
have his research gain the credibility it deserves, I would
be most happy, and I will discuss some of his findings
shortly. In fact, as those of you who have kept up with
my research know, if all I ever achieve in my work is to
aid in the creation of a vegetarian world, I will be most
happy. Being able to inspire people to honor all life so
that they can dance with the Divine is also high on my
list of priorities. Recently, I agreed to deal with the
Australian 60 Minutes television team. I did this in the
hope that they would do some solid investigative
journalism, to clear the media misinformation on the
deaths over the last three years, of three people associated
with the 21-day process. If I say that it is sad when our
loved ones die, people respond with why are you
attached to life when death does not exist as the spirit is

immortal and that changing bodies is just like changing clothes.

Don't you know that the time of our birth and death is between you and your God? On the highest level who is really responsible for life and death on this planet? If I say, should we blame a car manufacturer every time someone dies in a car accident, others say but three people died and someone should be held responsible. Car manufacturers and car dealers expect people to learn to drive, to follow driving guidelines, to drive safely and responsibly. A recent study done by the Centres for Disease Control and Prevention said that sedentary lifestyles and fast food diets are resulting in one in five Americans today being obese, and that this is killing 280,000 people in the U.S.A. each year. Are the fast food manufacturers responsible for this? Yet regardless of how responsibly we all act, as many now know, sometimes it is just our time to die.

Treating our body as a temple, acting impeccably and responsibly in every moment is part of the journey of self-4mastery, and if we all do that, then for any of us to take responsibility over the death of another, is like pretending we are the sun, rather than the sunshine of the sun. It is now the belief of many that each one of us has a time contract each life to be here, and when this is complete we leave either via accident, disease or, like the lamas we sit in meditation, and exit our body which then dies. Surely, it is time that we acted as responsible adults and took control over our lives and stopped looking to blame each other when our own choices create problems such as disease and even death. For any of us to take responsibility for another's choice is to undermine the very message of our work in the field of self mastery. Self-responsibility is the key to true inner and outer peace in this world, and some may say that blame perpetuates victim consciousness. Others may say that people die everyday and yes it is hard for those of us who loved them and miss them. In our grief we feel anger and denial and blame. In our sorrow we see life as limited, and in our ignorance we reject the very notion that the Divine One Within really is in charge. And in our arrogance we wish to prove to a non believing world, the existence of something that perhaps they are not yet ready to know. I say this because it was partly my own arrogance and also my naivete, that led me to accept the challenge put forward by 60 Minutes.

For years people have been telling me its impossible to do something that I have been doing for years. 28 years ago doctors told me that if I went vegetarian I would die from lack of protein but I didn't. 25 years ago doctors told me I could never have children but I did. 23 years ago doctors told me that having a home birth was dangerous and would risk the life of my child, but it didn't. 7 years ago doctors told me I couldn't heal my own cancer but I did. Now doctors tell me I will die if I do not eat food. Yes, it gets tiring listening to the same old fear and disbelief that comes from those who have not yet had the pleasure of experiencing their DOW, or who aren't prepared to move beyond limitation. And so I allowed myself to play the prove it to me game with 60 Minutes, lost my joy and became sincerely humbled.

My learning was invaluable. I must admit it was fascinating to be held in what felt like a POW camp with constantly changing rules, and I gained some wonderful insights! Particularly about the effects of sleep deprivation and carbon monoxide poisoning on the body when one isn't drinking, as I usually choose to do, to combat any negative effects of pollution, particularly when I travel. There is still so much I do not know about prana power and how it can nourish us fully as we exist in a modern day world, but as more of us live it and experience it, the more we understand.. Not eating and not drinking in a polluted environment was something the American founder of breatharianism, Wiley Brooks, had done in-depth research on before, but was not my field. Wiley had told me that he found it difficult to stabilize his weight when he was not drinking and not eating, and he felt it was due to the pollution and I never realized why, but now I do. Without the fluid to flush out the toxins, our body diverts precious energy to do this as it does when it has to digest food in the normal way. So I learnt personally that what Wiley had found is also true for me. Perhaps when we are more in tune with our DOW, we can go beyond even this. I feel that my recent media experiences are something that we can all learn from.

I found that we do not need to prove anything to anyone but ourselves, even though part of me would love pranic nourishment to be given acknowledgement as it could then be applied appropriately and really benefit many. Still, we all know that when we walk our talk and have a deep and profound experience no one can take that away from us. Yes it is unfortunate that although 60 Minutes were given all my research and findings plus 10 years of detailed scientific research by nuclear physicist Lu Zuyin, by their own admission none of this was read, and yes it is true that the interviewer decided to portray me as someone who was deluded. To this I responded.... What appears to be delusion to some is simply a preferable reality to another, for without our dreams and visions, humanity has no hope. Divine revelations come to those who sincerely ask to have them; this is the nature of the Higher Laws of Science that some call Universal Law. Only when humankind understands and applies these laws may peace, true unity and contentment reign permanently on earth. 60 Minutes were given a brilliant educational opportunity and decided not to take it, yet I am not interested in denigrating anyone except to say that in all my years of working with the media, I have come to understand that what is reported always reflects the consciousness of the journalist and their editor or producer. Nonetheless I have met some brilliant switched on and very enlightened journalists who operate with complete integrity and honour, and the German filmmaker Frieder Mayrhofer is one. Frieder has been following the progress of many people as they have been learning to live on light and even though various TV stations have been told of his work, most have been more interested in focusing on sensationalism rather than fact.

People ask me why I persevere with the media and to this I always say that it is my divine blueprint as a cosmic reporter to do this, as the media is one of the most powerful tools we have for planetary re-education today —provided it is used with honour and integrity and not for the sake of sensationalism. I think one of the problems of some of the less enlightened media is that they underestimate the intelligence of their audience. After the 60-Minute show went to air in Australia, they asked for feedback from their audience via a vote to the question Do you believe a person could live for six months on nothing but air and light? and 68% of the 1600 who called in actually said YES. The reason that I tell this story is because something magnificent is occurring on earth right now. People are having what I call divine experiences and what's more, many are now prepared to stand up and be counted.

So what exactly is all the controversy about my work? It seems that the some of the media in our world is convinced that my claim to be able to tune into the power of the Divine and live by its light is either fraudulent or crazy and deluded, even though the research has been done to prove that it is possible, provided people live a virtuous and spiritually enriching lifestyle.

To me a spiritually enriching lifestyle is a holistic lifestyle that allows us to be physically fit as we treat the body like a temple, emotionally fit as we treat ourselves and each other with love, honour and respect, mentally fit by being responsible for all our thoughts words and actions and applying and understanding the universal laws, and spiritually fit by aligning with, and experiencing the love, wisdom and power of the Divine One Within us—our DOW. So I would like to discuss Divine Power, how to experience it and also how to live our lives in alignment with the Divine Blueprint as for the past few months, I have been very focused in discussions and invitations to prove the existence of the Divine and tonight I would like to begin to lay the groundwork to do just that. For only when we have a direct experience of the Divine force in action can we truly surrender to divine will and serve in the unfoldment of the Divine Plan on earth. From this focus we will experience personal paradise and from this will come global paradise. American author Harold Sherman once said: "The more you depend on forces outside of yourself, the more you are dominated by them." To me freedom comes from detachment from the material world and a deep experience of the internal world of our DOW. Our DOW holds the key to our discovery of true happiness, health and wealth and our DOW is the common thread that binds and unites us all regardless of our beliefs.

I'd like to read you the opening paragraph to my new book Ambassadors of Light; We live in an age of magnificence-of prosperity and true joy and it only takes a recipe to tune us all in. What miracles are these that we have been given so much love, wisdom and power to use at our discretion?

Many of the Ambassadors of Light believe that we come as Gods to find the Gods that we are in physical earth form. Some say that God is like the sun. It feeds us, and keeps all our movies alive and Its nature can be nirvanic and tender.

When we swim in It, merge with It, feel It, allow It to love us as we remember It, miracles happen. Some call living without the need of food a miracle, yet our deepest and most nourishing sustenance comes from learning to dance with the Divine. In a recent interview in Switzerland, another servant of the Divine, the Lady Master Ching Hai was asked about proving the existence of God to people and she said How can I prove it to them? I don't want to. I'm not here to prove that God exists or doesn't exist. I just want to help you know God if you want to. She goes on to say that it is possible to experience God, if you want to, but for those who don't want to, that is fine too, and that's how I feel. For those who are willing to apply a little discipline in their daily lifestyle choice, for those who are willing to spend time in the silence of prayer and contemplation via meditation, for those who are willing to be the master of their body, mind and emotions, for those who are willing to put aside personal agendas and truly serve, for those who are willing to love unconditionally, for those who see their body as the temple for the Divine One Within to exist in the world of form—miracles will happen, and Holiness and true divinity will reveal itself. This is the scientific principle of Universal Law. No one can prove the existence of God except us, to us, for us. No one can give us the sincere desire to know who we truly are-beyond our mind, our emotions or our body.

Sincerity must come from deep within us, the longing to feel the oneness of creation must come from deep within us. Only we can find and experience our DOW and only our DOW has the power to unite and harmonize our inner and outer world. To those interested in the commonalties of science and the Divine—God, Allah, Brahma, are also names for what quantum calls the

Singularity. Yet while science continues to see spirit and matter as separate, scientists will not be able to fully understand the complexity of the quantum field. Qi is the essence of this field and Qi or DOW emissions defy normal scientific study which requires the observer to be detached from the experiment. Because of the nature of Qi, the observer and the observed are one and the same.

Just before I left Australia I received data which scientifically proves the reality of reincarnation. It involves an in-depth study of 2,600 children that was done by Ian Stevenson, a psychiatrist and professor dedicated to the scientific method, studying their claims of previous lives of which they had full recall. Working with Tom Schroder, an award winning journalist for the Washington Post they literally proved that the claims these children made are true by tracking down and their past life families and checking all the information given. Their work is now in the book *Old Souls : The Scientific Evidence for Past Lives* and is published by Simon & Schuster. In this book Tom Schroder tried to play the sceptic and disbeliever focusing only on fact, but as they found together these children had not only full recall, but birthmarks, birth defects, internal diseases, abnormalities of pigmentation, physique, posture, gesture and movements that can be tied to the subjects previous lives. Schroder says it was these facts that provided the science.

Even though the prestigious Journal of the American Medical Association had to admit that their work done over 35 years, contained evidence that would be very difficult to explain in any other way than reincarnation, and regardless of the massive amount of work in these two volumes, and the exhaustive amount of cross testing done, still the scientific community continues to ignore it. As Tom Schroder says "Because something challenges the accepted understanding of the world, it obviously cannot be true, and therefore is unworthy of consideration."

The earth is the center of the universe and that is that! How long must we bury our heads in the sand? Humanity must progress into a unified and harmonious existence— this is the nature of the divine dance we call evolution and we can only do this when we combine intelligence, with an openness and willingness to discerningly listen to new ideas and find the courage to adopt them if they are beneficial to our species. In depth research has been done on external Qi emissions but not enough on internal Qi radiation, except we do know that virtuous living, meditation, prayer, programming, diet and exercise directly influence internal Qi and its external radiation or emissions. The scientific community continues to ignore the work of the Qi Masters.

Similarly, the media, and the medical community continues to dismiss the work of the Light Ambassadors and our research into prana power which dovetails beautifully with Dr. Yan Xin's work, for Qi is DOW power in action. In my research, Qi emissions relate to the field of advanced bioenergetics and the higher light science, which I begin to cover in my autobiographical book *Our Camelot—The Game of Divine Alchemy*. We discuss it in greater depth in my new book *The Wizard's Tool Box*. Yes, it's great to now know that enough studies have been done to prove that magnetic field measurements coming from internal organs increase greatly when Qi is increased through the above lifestyle but this work now needs to be shared with the world so that all can benefit. Research has also been done on the effect of Qi in improving and regulating the function of the digestive system; how it improves the function of the endocrine system; how it affects our capacity to create changes in the muscular and skeletal systems; how it improves the functions of the respiratory system and the circulatory system; plus how it improves and regulates the functions of the nervous system, as well as the power that Qi has in adjusting skin temperature and controlling the body temperature center.

In eastern philosophy Qi is also called prana and it is known that the body's natural production of prana increases through the raising of the Kundalini energy via meditation and a yogic lifestyle. According to the Qi Masters, because Qi or prana runs on the neutrino level, it is very difficult to detect as Qi is what fills the 99% of space in each atom. The Qi Masters have proved that Qigong healing is also not just psychological. It has objective effects independent of the psychological dimension. For example, x-rays of a bone fracture before a Qi transmission, then an x-ray of a bone fracture after this transmission has shown how the fracture has been completely healed in a matter of hours or even minutes. Also it is known that Qi emissions do not lose their intensity over distance and can be directed by mind, will and intention, hence their effectiveness in distant healing. By moving their inner vision into the magnetic field of a patient, a Qi master can provide accurate diagnosis without actually seeing that patient, or being in the presence of that patient. Dr. Yan Xin was described as a contemporary sage by former President George Bush and his focus of research has long been on the benefits of applied Qigong into the areas of cancer and AIDS. As a result of attending his lectures, thousands of people have been cured of many major illnesses.

Like the Ambassadors of Light, Dr. Yan Xin encourages the respect for the old and care for those in need, while emphasizing the importance of a virtuous lifestyle and the value of love for others. Compassion, love and selfless service are key factors in the establishment of personal and global paradise as we enter a new millennium on earth, as is the respect and honoring of all life. Traditional Qigong theories hold that all things in the universe originate from Qi, that everything contains Qi, and that it fills the entire universe. This concurs with the Christian idea that God is omnipresent and omnipotent. A Qigong masters Qi emanations and power is closely related to his/her own physical, mental and emotional state at the time of the Qi transmission. In my recent experience with 60 Minutes, my weight loss of 5 kilos over 5 days occurred not only due to the natural water loss from the body, sleep deprivation and having to deal with pollution, but also due to my own emotional and mental state. Yes I felt annoyed at myself for allowing a media circus to take place around a sacred initiation, and trust people who did not have my interests at heart. And when we get frustrated, angry or lose our joy, we lessen our connection to our DOW and this interferes with our DOWs ability to nourish us. Arrogance, ego, fear, judgement and annoyance all inhibit the pranic flow and take us out of the Divine Dance Zone. So yes, the Light Ambassadors ability to be constantly fed by Qi or prana depends on our ability to maintain a high level of physical, emotional, mental and spiritual fitness can live on Qi alone for long periods of time and these fitness levels fluctuate according to what we are choosing to focus on in each moment.

According to the book *Qigong Scientific Exploration;* One may question how a person can live without food? First, the gastric and intestinal fluid of Qigong practitioners contain many nutrients. Second, everyone has nutrients stored in the body; yet most people do not how to transform and utilize them. Third, twenty or more days may pass without eating food, yet one can still be energized by absorbing self transformed high energy substances. It is not a question of eating, but rather of absorbing nutrients in a different manner. One can utilize the body's accumulated nutrition and transfer it to gastric and intestinal fluids for high quality nourishment. This also improves the digestive system. Qigong practitioners do not merely absorb nutrients through their mouths and noses.

They can use many other ways to absorb high energy substances for nourishment. Water, for instance, does not have to enter only through the mouth. Light does not have to enter only through our eyes (Like a plant that requires light photo-synthesis, light also has a function in our body.) A Qigong practitioner absorbs high energy substances from the universe that are unavailable to others.

In this manner one can eat less, or even not eat for a length of time and still maintain a high energy level. When the absorption of high energy substances is enhanced, one may go without food for a long period of time. That is why Qigong is an ideal way to improve the digestive system of the body. Traditional Qigong concerns itself with the effect of consciousness on an object and how the observer and the observed are connected, which is something traditional science has not yet accepted. Hence, the Qigong phenomena raises many questions for science which cannot be answered by current scientific theories. It has become my understanding, from my parallel research to the Qigong studies, that until scientists begin to experience their DOW, many answers to the mysteries of life, evolution and creation, will remain hidden from them. The Divine Dance is an experience, not a conceptual hypothesis and it can only be gained by a lifestyle that honors both intellect and intuition, head and heart. According to the scientists measuring Qigong emissions and studies on the Bigu state—that is not eating-many people in Bigu like myself, can live on less than 300 calories per day for years without any damage to their physical bodies.

In October 1987, Ding Jing, aged 10, went into the Bigu state and stayed there for over 6 years with a calorie intake of between 260 and 300 per day. We have found the same amongst the Light Ambassadors, and many continue to live very healthily on calorie intakes that are continuing to defy and challenge modern medical and scientific belief. Personally I have become healthier through Bigu and have proved to myself beyond doubt that my DOW is nourishing my body as have many other Ambassadors of Light. Medical science is slowly catching up with these ideas, for example, the August 27th edition of Science results of a research project by USA, Madison researchers Tomas A. Prolla and Richard Weindruch found that key genes that normally deteriorate with age continued to function in a youthful way when mice were underfed and from this they are now convinced that if people overeat they will accelerate the aging process. Halving the calorie content of the test mice diet doubled their lifespan. Other research shows that when people add daily meditation, regular exercise, positive mental and emotional attitudes, become vegetarian and practice loving rather than judging, their health and relationships improve dramatically. I am convinced after 28 years of personal research that all world health and world hunger related challenges can disappear with this change in lifestyle choice. Meditation stimulates altruism and the desire for unity and selflessness through service and my Ambassadors of Light book goes into great detail as to how we can redistribute the worlds resources to address current world hunger issues.

Regardless of how people react to this work, it has a valid place on the global stage that will, in time, be recognized and so the Qi practitioners like myself, will continue. Dr. Yan Xin (Shin) is one of the most respected and widely recognized Qi Masters in China and it is with his co-operation that such in depth studies on the benefits of Prana or Qi power have been conducted and shared with the world. Many people have spontaneously entered into the Bigu state as a result of being in his presence, and much research has been documented in the Chinese language. In fact over sixty books have been written covering his research into the power and benefits of Qi emissions. Professor Lu Zuyin's book is one of the first to be published in English and was only released in 1997 after a ten year period of research and experimentation. In 1987 I also began to record in my journals my conscious study and research on a) the power of internal Qi radiation, b) how our lifestyles can alter the levels of this radiation, and c) how to control our external fields of reality by controlling our Qi emissions internally and externally. The Qi masters say that Bigu is a state in which a person maintains a normal life without taking any food.

Standard Bigu means very little or no intake of water. Basic Bigu means only drinking water and juice. Non-standard Bigu means ingesting water, juice and occasionally juicy fruits and vegetable soups. The difference between the experience of the Light Ambassadors and those in the Bigu state is that we have sought this experience consciously by the practice of meditation and lifestyle choice that promote our becoming fit on all levels. Like myself, Dr Yan Xin, who I have not had the pleasure of meeting, has been guided to share this information with the world because of its benefits to humanity. Both of us recognize that major research still needs to be done into the Bigu phenomena and trust that as humanity focuses more on DOW power, that this will naturally come to pass. We present our research to the interested parties in the fields of science and medicine and trust that relevant studies will be done in time and the benefits will then be more widely shared. After completing the *Ambassadors of Living on Light* book which shares my own in depth research plus that of Austrian Dr. Karl Graninger who spent 20 years studying 23 people who lived without the need of food; I was given the Scientific Qigong Exploration manual, and hence my desire to bring this research to the attention of the world. Also, since I completed my research, as we have mentioned another person has died from exposure to the elements and slight dehydration while undergoing the 21-day process. Some would say she died as a result of not adhering strictly to the guidelines in my first book on this matter, Living on Light; others would say that her work was complete and she had come to the end of her contract and need to be here. Regardless of the whys, I cannot stress enough that we will continue to encourage all beings to take responsibility for their every thought, word and action in dealing with their own lives and the lives of others where appropriate. I must stress again that it is not necessary to undergo the 21-day process as many are now living on prana without undergoing this initiation.

However, if you are called from deep within to do this, then please act responsibly. Listen to your body, listen to your DOW and walk away, stop, if you get into difficulty. It is not important if we eat or don't eat. What is important is that we experience our DOW, and enjoy each moment in our lives in a way that benefits and honours all life. Yes it is part of my blueprint to bring this information to the world, yes it is true that I am free from the need to live on food (as we know it) and that my DOW does, has and will feed me. Yes it is also true that I was led into a field of research, as a result of my experience with my DOW, that may have many wonderful global benefits for health and hunger related issues. Yes it is true that whether people believe this or not, there are those who have experienced the power of the Divine enough to know, that when we truly have experienced something we cannot deny it, even though many others may not believe. Like the Master Ching Hai, I have no desire to convince the world of anything, only to share what I feel to be some most interesting research as it is my divine service to do so. Self-responsibility, kindness, compassion, selfless service and altruistic behavior are all keys to the Divine dance floor. As the Indian author A. Parthasarathy once said: Modern civilized men without self-development are but intelligent savages living in spiritual slums. In a moment, I would like to complete this evening with something very practical. Yes, it is a program that if applied by all will guarantee religious unification, but it is also a program to allow us all to enjoy more of the Divine Dance of life. Just our commitment and desire to find and enjoy the evidence of Holiness will indeed change our world regardless of what we all call our God. The evidence of Holiness comes to us automatically when we use the following program:

Before we begin let me just share the following with those of you unfamiliar with the power of prayer and programming:

Researching neuro-science has established a state called plasticity which is our brain's inherent capacity to change. This is actually mirroring the universal law of change and adaptation. The human brain constantly designs new patterns, new combinations of nerve cells and neurotransmitters in response to new input and stimuli. Each individual has the potential to rewire the brains neural map and reconfigure it in a manner more conducive to producing the life they are looking for. Some of you may wish to utilize the programs listed throughout the Ambassadors of Light book and remember that when we ask we will receive. This is universal law. Programming utilizes thoughts, words and prayers and has the ability to create new software for our bodies—

the hardware—to run more effectively in life. When DOW power awakens en masse the way it now is, changes automatically happen. Everyone has this power available to them—in the same quantities—we just access it with different regularity and in different quantities. DOW Power is not restricted by our races, religions, cultures or our beliefs. It is like a hidden source of energy that when recognized, connected with, experienced and allowed to flow unimpeded through our bodies, brings many miracles to our lives. As my friend and colleague, Louix Dor Dempriey says in his book *Dawn of Enlightenment: Divinity* reveals itself from within the self, where it lies dormant until such time as the soul is ready and willing to externalize it. There are four qualities necessary to liberate the soul: desire, faith, willingness and obedience. Of the four, obedience is the last to which the ego personality will succumb. It is not enough to read all the right books and quote all the great sages. The divine laws of cause and effect must be obeyed. Thank you Louix.

The evidence of these laws is everywhere on our planet if only we choose to look. So is the evidence of Holiness which appears in different ways to different people. And yet it is not our different beliefs that stop us from experiencing Holiness—it is our lack of deep desire. Without desire, without intention and without vision, the evidence of the Supreme Splendour remains hidden from us all. Those who have found and experienced the evidence of Holiness often become the Ambassadors of Light. So the following program is simple and not to be underestimated in its power. It is one that I have developed for the sole purpose of religious unification on earth and to allow individuals to really experience the divine if it is their sincere desire to do so. For those of you present who desire this, let us close our eyes and pray and program together: I will share the program once to familiarize you with it, then you can repeat it after me. I now surrender into the experience of the revelation of paradise on a personal and global level. I ask the universe to bring me the evidence of Holiness and Godliness and graciousness and divinity in such a manner that I am permanently moved beyond doubt. I now choose to forgive all those who have ever harmed me or my ancestors. I ask for forgiveness for all that I have ever done that has created harm. I now enter the new millennium with the love of my God in my heart, accepting and honoring of all who honor life. So it is. So it is. So it is.

CHAPTER 14

"10,000 Now Living on Light"

An update by Jasmuheen: so much has happened over the last 5 years since the Living on Light phenomena hit the global stage. With over 10,000 individuals now allowing the Divine to feed them, plus many more in the Qigong community who exist in the state of Bigu, the idea that the Divine can not just love, guide and heal us, but also feed us, is slowly being accepted.

As the ability to live on light is completely related to a person's daily lifestyle, the actual 21-day initiation has become passé as more and more holistic living practitioners find themselves eating light.

Our research has found that the long term practice of meditation, prayer, programming, vegetarian diet, exercise, service, silence in nature and the use of Mantras and devotional songs, expand a person's consciousness, thus allowing them to exist in the zone of the Divine where so much more than normal reality is possible. We call this 8-point program the Luscious Lifestyles Program—or L.L.P.—and it is basically designed to tune people into the frequency where Living on Light is no longer a miracle.

Due to the power of the media, we have been able to talk about Divine Power, the Source that feeds us, to more than 6 million in less than 3 years, although the media has not always been supportive.

In 1996, shortly before this book was published in the

German language, a young man went into a coma during the process, was admitted to hospital, woke up and was on the road to recovery when he had an epileptic fit, fell over and hit his head on the back of the bed and died.

Two years later an Australian woman refused to stop the initiation even though her care giver recommended she do so. She also fell into a coma and was subsequently taken off life support by her family, when the doctors found her to have internal damage from dehydration and other issues. Her care giver and his wife were later jailed for negligence. In late 1999, another Australian woman living in Scotland died when she chose to ignore the guidelines in this book, stopped eating and drinking, traveled for a few days, and ended up collapsing from exhaustion and dying from exposure to the elements.

While I have had no dealing with any parties involved, the blame of their deaths landed on my doorstep as some in the world felt that the Living on Light reality is impossible and unsafe. The fact that in 1999, 280,000 Americans died from over-eating is to them, irrelevant. The fact that after alcohol and tobacco, meat eating is the third biggest killer in the western world is also to many irrelevant.

Yet to me every human being must take responsibility for their own life and act accordingly. If we live a healthy lifestyle through food choices we can live longer, and prana is a food choice—not a common one yet, but however it is a valid and healthy one and thousands now attest to this.

Regardless of whether Living on Light and being nourished by prana is socially acceptable or not, the fact remains for thousands it is now a preferable lifestyle and pretending that it is not possible so that non-believers can feel more comfortable in their reality, is not going to happen.

For those wishing to be nourished by the Divine I can

only urge you to prepare as well as possible by following the Get Fit for Prana guidelines. Also note that the 21-day initiation does not necessarily guarantee that the Divine will feed you, only your daily practice of the Luscious Lifestyles Program can do that. We also recommend that you only do the 21-day process if it makes your heart truly sing. Like many ancient spiritual initiations, the 21-day process is designed to test your trust and faith, and unless you have clear inner guidance with your Divine One Within, your DOW, I personally recommend that you do not do it and wait until you do trust this inner voice 100 percent. You also need to have a very strong mind/body connection where you can listen to all the subtle signals and nuances that the body constantly displays in communicating with its Master.

These days I tend to recommend the Germans' approach to Living on Light, as it is long term and sensible and does not involve any difficult initiation. In this reality, for example, they set themselves a 5-year plan to slowly prepare their physical, emotional and mental bodies, while also conditioning their family and friends to this new intended reality. For example, year 1—no more meat; year 2—become a vegan, no more dairy products; year 3—raw food only; year 4—fruit only; year 5—juices only; year 6—prana only. During this 5 year period, they also plan to exercise and meditate regularly and become as finely tuned as possible, allowing them to expand their consciousness to live permanently in the Divine airwaves.

In 1999, I completed my book "Ambassadors of Light-World Health and World Hunger Project" which takes the Living on Light discussion on to the global stage re health and hunger issues. Full of research and statistics, it provides a wonderful argument for global vegetarianism and resource sustainability.

While the personal and global benefits of pranic nourishment are obvious, Living on Light is still not a sociably acceptable lifestyle and many light eaters choose to be very selective regarding who they share this information with. Also as you can't hide the fact that you do not eat from family and friends, you need to realize that to many, living free from the need for food as we know it is an absolutely impossible reality, yet to those who have experienced the power of the Divine, miracles happen daily.

Living on Light and the 21-day process will not offer a quick fix to health or life problems, nor is it an easy road to enlightenment. Only what we fill each moment of our day with can determine this and while this reality attracts spiritual warriors who accept themselves as their own Masters, we can only ask that you treat yourself and this initiation with the utmost responsibility and respect.

I would also like to note that over the last 3-4 years we have been dealing and negotiating with various Research Institutes to try and bring in a more scientific understanding of the power of prana and its ability to nourish our cells and not just our souls. Unfortunately, due to lack of funding we have had minimal success with this. However, we are currently negotiating with a major US institute and plan to undergo in-depth testing in 2002.

Once again we stress, do not do this 21-day initiation process unless it really speaks to every fibre of your being and makes your heart truly sing, for this is not an initiation that will guarantee Living on Light. It is an initiation that will allow you to dance on a deeper level with your Divine Self and provided you are physically, emotionally, mentally and spiritually fit then you, like many thousands of others, may experience the true gifts of this initiation on many, many levels.

Remember that this is the path of self mastery, and unless you have complete 100 percent trust in your Divine inner voice, and good clear communication with your body, then once more we recommend you take the less controversial path for Living on Light – the 5 year-plan. The main focus needs to be on our lifestyle so that we may be in the correct frequency where this is possible.

The L.L.P. 8-STEP Program includes the following points:

- Daily Meditation
- Prayer
- Programming
- Light vegetarian diet
- Exercise
- Service
- Time in silence in nature
- Use of mantras, chanting and devotional song.

In Biofield Science, every being has the potential to enjoy YOUR BODY FITNESS.

This is obvious when we see it for people are happy with their love health and wealth quotient and they enjoy passion and purpose and good relationships with life.

Wishing your path of great joy, harmony and happiness.

Namaste, Jasmuheen.

CHAPTER 15

Testimonials of Pranic Nourishment

Below I reproduce experiences of pranic nourishment and a justification for it.

Food for Thought (if not for Eating)
by Meghan Stevens

There would be no doubt that if someone tried most of the siddhis, be it walking through fire (the easiest— although some still end up in the burn ward of the local hospital), stopping one's heart beat, sitting in snow all night while drying wet blankets on one's back, or being buried alive without air, they would come to harm.

Yogis dedicate their entire lives to the practices that often, as a side effect, allow them to perform unusual disciplines of mind and body. Along a similar vein, in theory it is possible for many people to run fast enough to win a gold medal at the Olympics, but would anyone attempt it unless they had trained day in, day out, month in month out, year in year out?

It is important to understand that the training for the ability to be able to survive without eating is not, to stop eating. Similarly, no one suggests that the training to be able to be buried alive without oxygen is not to stop breathing.

These abilities involves decades of advanced yoga meditation practices. Therefore, it is not reasonable to suppose that anyone could undergo a short training period and then stop eating.

A Breatharian Experience

The Breatharian experience, like many special states, may arise spontaneously. I have experienced the Breatharian state to some extent for a very short time. I state absolutely that it did not involve any hunger, hallucination, weakness or ill health.It happened to me naturally, at a mountain ski resort. The prana was so strong in mountain air, each breath was exhilarating but it was more than the prana, it was my physical and psychic response to a specific time and place.

I felt no urge to eat or drink and sipped only small amounts of water and nibbled even smaller amounts of food. Each day I ate less until it was literally only a mouthful at each meal. This was not because I was trying to fast but a mouthful filled me. My hunger disappeared, my energy levels soared and I skied all day everyday. I felt and looked vibrantly healthy and did not lose weight! This continued for a week. Unfortunately, as soon as I left the environment, the spell was broken. It was a naturally occurring "spell"—one of the very occasional "enlightenment" experiences, and can not later be replicated.

If you insist on checking whether you have this siddhi, it's important to remember that if you feel hungry, become unwell or lose weight, it is a definite sign that you must not continue and that you must go back to a normal diet.

My Experience... An Unfinished Story
Dr. Juergen Buche , N.D., MI, N.H.C., Phy.D.

When I first read about Breatharianism (also called INEDIA) in Viktoras Kulviskas' marvelous book "Survival into the 21st Century", it took years for me to realize that the very first line of his chapter on "Breatharianism" which reads: "NOT FOR EVERYBODY" was more than 'pregnant with meaning'.

In summer of 1993, I was slowly returning North from Miami, Florida on my yacht "Angerica II" with only me onboard. When departing Miami, I decided that I would do a fast. I certainly did not set myself a time limit but it seemed appropriate. Off and on, during the past eight years, I had fasted often, mostly a day or two at a time, but fairly often. I had developed a decent conscience regarding food but felt that I needed to detoxify more seriously than I had before. There were also certain 'afflictions' which I had endured for a very long time such as not being able to smell for over twenty years. My taste was naturally also severely restricted. Just hold your nose and try to taste something other than strictly salty or sweet or bitter (the primary taste sensations of the tongue).

One thing scared me a bit. Every authority on fasting advocates the essential need for rest, inactivity, calm and serenity. Life as a single-hander on a large yacht may be serene but it is anything BUT tranquil, inactive and restful!

Nevertheless, I proceeded to sail North along the Intracoastal Waterway, for over 1,000 miles, day in and day out, for three weeks, until I arrived at Elizabeth City in North Carolina. By that time I smelled whatever you placed under my nose. A miracle? Not at all. I had simply detoxified and cleared my sinus cavities. I had also lost quite a bit of weight and looked a bit drawn and haggard. The sight of me was probably not pretty because, when my wife and brother arrived to accompany me on the remaining trip to Montreal, Canada, they gave me curious looks and expressed concern over my appearance. That, of course, is to be expected if you do an uncontrolled fast. Later, in this dissertation, you will discover what I mean by 'controlled'.

Some people think they are fasting when they take no food for 12 hours. Hogwash! Some believe they are fasting when they abstain from solids and take only juices of some kind. Hogwash! Fasting means taking no food other than water. Some people advocate not drinking ANY water. I cannot support that approach. As long as the human organism is still toxic, there is a need to eliminate dying cells (result of catabolism), cellular refuse, discharged lymph, old fecal matter and undesirable substances such as toxic mucus, liver and kidney stones and gravel and many other waste products we cannot even start defining. While the body is not eating, there is a lot of house cleaning going on, both on a physical level as well as a mental and emotional level. Only later will such house cleaning spill over to the spiritual level. As you can see, there are many theories about fasting.

To continue my narrative...

During this voyage, I continued drinking at least one quart (one liter) of water early in the morning but very little during the day. Just enough to quench my thirst when needed. Invariably, I discovered that I had a short bowel movement (usually quite liquid) about 20 minutes after my morning drink. I did not mix this drinking water with anything whatsoever. The 'diarrhea' served as an excellent eliminative process. Long-term fasters usually start developing bad breath, disagreeable body odors and a variety of cleansing reactions that could be a bit overpowering for some bystanders. In my case, I perspired profusely throughout the day and did not develop any disagreeable cleansing reactions. This perspiration probably also initiated large losses of salt, minerals and trace minerals and I would not be surprised if some of my haggardness was due to this very reason. Today, I would mix my drinking water with maybe 1/4 sea water and that I would count on to replenish my missing minerals.

Although I had no adverse cleansing reactions, other fasters might have many and severe ones, too. I wished I had done a few liver cleanses before starting such a fast because several liver cleanses, three months apart, should get rid of all stones, gravel and crystals in the gall bladder and liver and thus should eliminate most cleansing reactions. A kidney cleanse and parasite cleanse are also most helpful but not mandatory. I took no medication or supplementation of any kind and do not recommend that this be done during a serious fast.

The day after I arrived at Elizabeth City, I started eating again. You'll never guess how! With Kentucky-fried chicken! Usually, authorities recommend that you start drinking orange juice, sparingly, and slowly graduate to more solid foods. I did not get sick, throw up nor did I reject such junk food! Mind you—it was just chicken—nothing else. So, at least I observed proper naturopathic food combining practices! (smile).

At that time I still had the notion that one needs protein to build muscle and to survive. Today, I know otherwise. You ARE what you THINK you are and any limitations between your ears become your very own and cry out for acceptance and expression in reality!

Thought forms are VERY powerful. If you 'KNOW' you must age—well, you will! Today, I WOULD break by fast (start eating again) on fresh fruit juices and would eat fruit only for at least a week until I could eat a raw (pesticide-loaded) vegetable salad. That's if I wanted to eat again! If you feel like it you might as well become a Breatharians at that point, that's the time to do it. I didn't then—but now the picture is different!

The one and lasting impression I had from that 3-week experience was that, after the third day, all feelings of hunger and all dependencies on food utterly disappeared. The liberating feeling of knowing that Cosmic Life Essence can and did and will sustain me for

undefined periods is wonderful. The clarity of mind one
develops during a complete fast is awesome. The breath
rate slows to under five per minute (what's yours now?)
and the heart rate is well below 60 (check yourself now)
—and yes, I worked hard throughout my fasting period.
I noticed no diminution of strength, no headaches and
no feelings of despair or anxiety. Off and on, there was
a certain queasiness in the stomach area, possibly a
certain adjustment of blood sugar levels and
transmutations of certain elements to replenish missing
trace elements and due to the liver starting to use stored
fat or glycogen to convert to glucose to feed the brain. I
drank my urine throughout the day to keep hormones
at an acceptable level and to augment my energy.

During this fast, conducted in the height of summer, I
lost a great deal of liquids and also a lot of minerals and
trace minerals through perspiration not through
urination. Drinking my urine was the only thing that
saved me from demineralization. If you have the slightest
queasiness about drinking your own Water of Life and
you perspire at all—then you MUST supply yourself with
necessary macro minerals and trace minerals until your
body has acquired the ability to transmute available
minerals into necessary unavailable minerals and
elements. This it does eventually, mostly from the
nitrogen of the air. The ideal intermediate source, for
several weeks, should be from sea vegetation, not from
land mineral deposits. One product has not only all of
the minerals and trace elements but also all the vitamins,
enzymes, and amino acids known to man. This is Kelp.
One ounce a day (two teaspoons) is sufficient and it will
not re-awaken the digestive processes because, being
totally natural and organic, it starts being assimilated
into your body as you retain it in your mouth for a minute
or so. Then swallow it. Once your body knows how to
transmute, under the solicited guidance of the Great

Cosmic Universal Source (via affirmations), then you can slowly cut back in the intake of Kelp. Your body will tell you when it is time to cut back. Know that sustenance comes from God, not from food. Food is but the catalyst that triggers the body to conduct certain processes and actions.

The foregoing is not at all remarkable but, I assure you, it is quite significant to me for several reasons that will become apparent as we continue together our journey into the fascinating realm of "Breatharianism".

Oh, by the way—in case you are wondering—not more than a week after my 3-week total fast, when I started to eat like a normal 'civilized' human again, I totally lost my sense of smell again.

Update 11 October, 2001: Where am I now—how have I evolved during the past few years and what is my present outlook regarding Breatharianism?

Basically, I eat (frugally) in the winter because the absence of sun makes it impossible for me to any long term fasting. I get skinny and haggard. But starting in the spring, when the sun comes out and I can take sun baths, I eat more and more frugally. I start TASTING small morsels of food instead of filling my gut with food. In essence, by then I have lost my addiction to food. I don't advertise this at all—even to my best friends— because everyone with whom I speak of this thinks I am crazy. So, consequently, I can't help keep this to myself. By preference, starting mid-April, I take one teaspoon of powdered kelp with a gulp of spring water everyday— sometimes I forget to eat even this little food. I drink of my own 'water of life' several times a day and have an almost liquid quick bowel movement every morning— cellular waste—that's all it is—but it gets washed out via the intestines. I drink several glasses of spring water in the morning, upon arising, to trigger this quick internal housecleaning. Sometimes, I have a glass of wine and find it very cleansing. Champagne would be better but I don't relish the headache.

Yes, I miss the companionship and pleasure that comes from human interaction during meals. I can watch people eat around me without any discomfort whatsoever and I delight in seeing and feeling my own liberation as compared to those who eat to live and live to eat. When you have looked at all the frightening Mad Cow Disease literature, as I have, then you are not at all sorry to be in the process of giving up eating. It is really easy when you KNOW (not think) that all sustenance comes from the Great Source of All There Is. When you carry an abundant supply of love and unload it on everyone and everything you come in contact with— then eating is such an unnecessary habit. Once you know how good it feels not having to detoxify, not having to eliminate those deadly toxins, not having to deal with choices of food and supplements, when health is the birthright you have claimed for yourself—then not eating, or at least eating VERY frugally, is the best ticket to liberation you could have bought for your own salvation. Ascension is only a stone throw away—and achievable.—J.B.

For several years now, I have explored the lives of people who, according to written accounts, have 'lived on air'. Some are historical Breatharians and others, like Dr. Barbara Moore and Jasmuheen are contemporaries.

There is also mounting evidence that biological transmutation is a fact—not only for plants but for humans as well. Kervan, often referred to in Christopher Bird's excellent book "The Secret Life of Plants", has done much to prove that plants have no trouble transmuting one element into another. If you look at the molecule of chlorophyll and that of hemoglobin, then you will see readily why the blood of plants (chlorophyll) is practically identical to human blood, with only one major difference—the nucleus. In plants it is magnesium and in humans it is iron. Is it really such an enormous stretch of an imagination to conclude that humans transmute chlorophyll into hemoglobin—practically instantly? And why is it that one can remove ALL the blood in an alley dog's body, fill it with diluted seawater and observe a healed, peppy, healthy dog just hours afterwards? And the seawater in this body does not remain as seawater of course—it turns into regular but healthier blood.

And what if transmutation can be directed and controlled by thought or affirmations? Why can we not make that quantum jump in consciousness? I tell you why—it is called brainwashing. We have been told all our life that food is ABSOLUTELY essential for life. But that is not necessarily so. If one person can go without food then all persons should be able to do this. So, what makes the difference? THINKING MAKES IT SO!

Medical Giants Speak on the Source of Life...

In the first quarter of this century, there existed a number of renowned doctor/scientists who were true humanitarians. Those were the medical giants that medicine could have built upon and learnt from but it never happened. Who, today, has heard of Dr. Henry Lindlahr, Dr. Rocine, Dr. Tilden, Dr. John Christopher, or even Dr. Bernard Jensen who was their student and is still alive today at age 88.

These illustrious giants advocated a natural approach to medicine, one tempered with patience and perseverance. They all had an excitingly fresh viewpoint of a LARGER medicine, a medicine that encompassed religion, science and humanities.

Listen to what Dr. Lindlahr had to say in his 1914 book "Natural Therapeutics—Dietetics, Volume III" page

50..."[Our] conception regards life as the primary force of all forces coming from the great central Source of all intelligence and creative power. This force, which permeates, heats and animates the entire created universe, is the expression of the "divine will", the "Logos", the "word" of the Great Creative Intelligence. Our sun is one of the millions of power stations for the distribution of this divine energy which sets in motion the whirls the ether [vortices] the electric [vibrational] corpuscles and ions that make up the different atoms and elements of matter. ...This intelligent energy can have but one source—the one and only Source of all life, intelligence and creative will in this universe. If this supreme intelligence would withdraw its energy ... the entire universe would disappear in a flash of a moment.

From this it appears that crude matter, instead of being the source of life and of all its complicated mental and psychical phenomena is but an expression of the Life Force, itself a manifestation of the Great Creative Intelligence which some call God, others Nature, the Oversoul, Brahma, Prana, the Great Spirit, and so forth, each according to his best understanding. It is this Supreme Intelligence and power, acting in and through every atom, molecule and cell in the human body, which is the true healer, the vis mediatrix naturae, which always endeavors to repair, to heal, and to restore (perfection). All that the physician can do is to remove obstructions and establish normal conditions within and around the patient, so that the "healer within" can do His work to the best advantage.

This life force is the primary source of all energy—that from which all other kinds and forms of energy are derived. It is independent of the body and of food and drink [just] as the electric current is independent of the glass bulb and the carbon thread through which it manifests as heat and light.

As you can see, the true historical doctors all had a healthy respect for a higher source of life. They were not tired prescription writers. They needed no referral to other 'specialists' who never knew the patient. The likes of Lindlahr knew how to assist the body and mind to normalize with a minimum of interference. I, Dr. Buche, have learned immensely from those medical giants!!!

As Kulviskas says: "There is a beautiful simplicity in this [Breatharian] approach. It enables one to get away from the gross and intoxicating nature of food which leads the average person to spend at least one third of his or her lifetime in the unconscious state of sleep and the rest of it in a stupor of unproductive, demoralizing labor."

This seems only too true. Have you watched TV lately, specially in the morning? The whole spiel is geared to cooking, food preparation and eating while pushing dietary products, all of which are processed and adulterated. In almost 15 years of Naturopathic praxis I have had only a handful of SERIOUS patients who have undertaken conscientious changes in diet and life style- for a while. None so far have expressed even remote interest in undertaking a practice such as Breatharianism in order to achieve a worthwhile goal. As a matter of fact, most patients visit me only to see what bad habits they can get away with while keeping their present illusionary life style. As Ponce de Leon was looking in vain for the Fountain of Youth, my patients, almost without exception, are forever looking for a silver bullet, the proverbial snake oil, that will cure all their ills but, if you please, without any effort on their part!!!

I have come to the conclusion that a therapist, a doctor, a practitioner can advise anything—and patients will follow blindly—as long as he/she does not impinge on the patient's dietary habits. EATING is so engrained, so pleasantly intoxicating, seemingly so NECESSARY in the eyes of everybody you see around you, that the mere reference to Breatharianism evokes smiles of pity and raises eyebrows of consternation if not outright condemnation and ridicule. And all that is easily provoked without the slightest hint at study or learning or—heaven forbid—practising a day of fasting—on the part of the one who raises those eyebrows in wonder at your evident insanity.

It is not enough to try to go without food. You must have a pretty good idea about the underlying reasons why you want to do without food. Are you doing this to gain notoriety or fame? Are you doing this because you are ill and want to heal, to regenerate, to rejuvenate? Are you properly prepared to actually draw from the great Universal Source the required sustenance to not only stay alive but to thrive in exquisite health and abundance?

I found that daily affirmations are an absolute necessity in order to reinforce the paradigm of self-sufficiency with the SELF being the almighty I AM resident within you. I affirm, with my heart center firmly engaged: "I AM limitless Love. I am the perfect manifestation of the omnipotent and benevolent power of the universe that sustains me from day to day regardless of whether I eat or not. I AM continually renewed in all respects, spiritually and emotionally balanced and I AM protected from all negative influences. I AM the perfect expression of divine and limitless Love."

The above affirmation will sustain you and protect you. Have no fear and dare to be different.

One other important ingredient, in my opinion, is to practise 'Inspirational Pranayama' in conjunction with the above affirmations. This is a simple breathing exercise that allows you to consciously tune into the Universal

Cosmic Supply and withdraw, at will, all the sustenance you wish. I call it 'square breathing'. It is extremely powerful to tune into the Universal Substance, prana, and consciously utilize this invisible, all-pervading, life-preserving, rejuvenating, primordial substance.

1. Sit comfortably, straighten you back and empty your lungs completely.
2. Start by inhaling completely to the count of four (seconds).
3. Retain your breath to the count of four.
4. Exhale completely to the count of four.
5. Keep your lungs empty to the count of four.
6. Repeat 2-5 ten times once a day or more often if desired.
7. Increase the count by 1 second each week (don't be in a rush even if this appears simple).
8. When the going gets rough (maybe at 10 seconds a leg) stay at that level until it is easy.
9. When taking a breath chant "Sooooo".
10. When exhaling, chant "Hummmmmm".

So, now you are on your way to become an accomplished Breatharian. Good for you! Can you estimate how much time, effort and money is wasted day in and day out—on eating and preparing food? Hardly! Eating is a very bad habit, it seems. People simply eat themselves to death. Experiments with rats have proven beyond a shadow of a doubt that halving their food intake doubles their life span.

Some Interesting Questions for Aspiring Breatharians...

Some interesting questions an aspiring Breatharian needs to find answers for are these:

"Can a person live without any food? For weeks, months, years? Is this for me?"

"Is nutrition derived from food or does it really come from the Universal Essence?"

"Is a radical departure of traditional 'religious' spiritual values a necessity?"

Other questions are secondary but stimulating just the same...

"How long can a detoxified person stay under water? 4 minutes, 10 minutes, an hour?"

It has never been tried—why not experiment a bit, or maybe a lot? Naturally, there will be a long period of transition.

The length of transition to true Breatharianism depends on the faster's belief system, his/her prime intent to become a Breatharian, his/her inherent constitution, his/her will to follow through with the required discipline, the amount of outside interference and his/her resistance to it, availability of sunshine and tranquility, the company he/she keeps and the amount of spiritual assistance that can be called upon and be sustained from the heavenly realms. Eventually, the Breatharian must learn to live with him/herself without support from society and re-learn certain concepts (and I quote from Leonard Orr's book: "The Common Sense of Physical Immortality"...)

"Why not have your laugh last and last?"

"Death is a useless custom, a bad habit."

"Death is a grave mistake."

"Visionary ideas may seem strange at first but they may save your live!"

"People value their bad habits more than their bodies."

"People value their false religions more than the living temple of God (their bodies)."

"Achieving physical immortality may be easier and more fun than your think."

"If you can't take it with you—don't go!"

"Death and taxes are no longer certain in life—they are now negotiable."

"Those who think they know what is right are particularly irritating to those of us who do!"

...and finally, the one I like a lot: "Dying is no way to live!"

One more reason to be a Light Eater:

In roughly two years and a few months from now, there is a distinct likelihood that a giant comet, four times the size of earth, will stream into our planetary system and wreak havoc as it has done every 3657 years.

When that happens, the catastrophic changes are so severe that eating as usual is just not feasible. Anyone who has had a history of fasting will fare much better than those who 'live to eat'. Those who are Light Eaters (Breatharians) will be able to cope infinitely better of course and can teach others, by their example, that sustenance as we know it, does not get derived from food but from cosmic prana (energy).

I will say no more, nor try to convince you one way or the other. The following links will either convince you or make you shudder or make you smile. In either case, any of these links will provide WEEKS of fascinating reading and might even save your life.

CHAPTER 16

An Awakening

Rev. Susan Skadron testifies:

I want you to know that I have been through an awakening. This has been an ordeal of great torment for me. I can't even remember everything that happened. It seems as though I experienced a spiritually induced psychotic break, and am aware of many things that were so disturbing that I can hardly be conscious of it!

It seems that I have been through such an ordeal that my personality influence has entirely disappeared. This means that spirit is running this body, and there are no illnesses left. I am aware that there are many people who can use the information that is coming through me now.

I have been through a 24-day water fast during this ordeal, and had no ill effects of any kind. This was very disturbing for me, because I was told that I was now Breatharian, and I believed that this meant that I would be without food for the rest of my life. This was actually fine physically, but emotionally it was upsetting, to say the least!

I found that the emotionally addictive relationship with food had disappeared. After this period, I was guided to start adding fruit juice to the water. I was so thrilled that I could have lemon and lime in my water that I no longer had any hunger influence.

It is important to know that my work continued without interruption during this entire period, even though I was severely psychologically disturbed. I had plenty of energy, and found that very little sleep was needed. I feel that I have been through such a disturbing period that I now have great news to share!

There has been such an awakening that I am able to teach food alchemy. This means that food is used in such a way as to build life force, without ever entering the digestive tract. This means that every food is completely digested while still in the mouth, and it entirely evaporates there. The life force is released from the food and is used for healing the body.

This is so important to teach, because one can literally eat all day without ever having a full belly! It requires complete detoxification, and I will be teaching this to everyone who shows the slightest interest. It appears that I have quite a full life ahead of me, as many people will want to know how to eat without weight gain of any kind.

Please know that this is as surprising to me as it is to you. I have been taught by my own Consciousness. This is happening all day and night. I am being trained to teach food alchemy using ayurvedic principles of ascorbate and aspartic energy. Please know that when combined properly and potentiated to a great degree, they become so powerful that it makes it possible to eat anything.

I have been allergic to chocolate ever since I ate some in childhood and was later told it was poisoned. I got quite ill from that, and never recovered. This has been true for most foods in my life, and I was on a severely restricted diet for the last 10 years. Now I find I can eat literally anything without any repercussions.

Please know that this has been such an ordeal that I have not been in touch with many who could not hear this until now. However, please know that I am here now, in a very different form, and am happy to be available for this teaching.

CHAPTER 17

Qigong Master Qinyin on Energized Fasting and Detoxification

Sigrid McLaughlin talks to Qigong Master Qinyin:

When I first heard of an extraordinary Qigong Master recently arrived from China, I had been doing Qigong for almost three years under the guidance of Dr. Hu from Berkeley. Qi-gong means literally life energy (qi or ch'i; the Indian prana, or Japanese ki) work or the benefits from persistent practice (gong or kung).

If you are healthy, the qi is plentiful and clear, and flows smoothly like a calm stream. It is an energy that permeates everything, including animals and plants, mountains and oceans, our earth (Gaia) and the universe. For the individual human being qigong means working with life energy to prevent its pollution, stagnation, and blockages, and to balance yang and yin aspects of this energy. Yang means the more male, positive, forceful, sun-like qualities, yin the more female, negative, soft, cooling, moon-like qualities. The result of practicing qigong is an improvement in the harmony and health of our body and mind/spirit.

Qigong uses healing postures, movements, breathing techniques and meditation to reach the goal of self-healing. The exercises are practiced daily, from twenty to forty minutes, and there are techniques for every age and physical condition, done standing, seated, or lying down. It empowers the practitioner to rely on himself and be responsible for his own health.

Qigong is as ancient as the beginnings of Chinese culture, probably going back to the animal dances of ancient Chinese shamans in the second and first millennium before Christ. Later Daoist and Buddhist philosophy influenced the meditative practices of Qigong, because both spirit and body need to be cultivated equally- an equivalent of our "sound mind in a sound body."

Master Qinyin came to the United States with an invitation to present her qigong system at the Second World Congress of Qigong in San Francisco in 1997. Her success there gave her the honor of "Distinguished Faculty" and "an alien with extraordinary ability"(Immigration Service) which entitled her to stay in the United States. Prior to this, she had been elected to be one of the elite members of the Chinese Qigong society (an honor which 1000 people achieve out of more than a billion Chinese), hailed as "little heavenly master Zhang" by the former chairman of the Chinese Qigong Research Association, Mr. Zhenhuan Zhang. Since then she achieved various honors and awards in the United States. When I learned of her existence and her new system of practices that resulted in astounding healings in China I decided to do her training.

My first surprise was that this master is a young and beautiful woman brimming with energy, not the white-haired, wrinkled old woman I had expected. The exercises were easy for me (I am sixty year old) except one; and the results were astounding. I have kept doing these practices almost daily, and will continue, as I notice their beneficial influence on my mind and body. I decided that it would be of great benefit to everyone in the United States to learn her techniques. She agreed to this interview to share more about herself and her system.

The Interview

McLaughlin: How did you get involved with Qigong in China?

Qinyin: I was born a sickly child in Han Zhou, in southern China. To help me survive, my maternal grandmother, a pious Buddhist, taught me to sit with her in meditation when I was three. Of my family I was the only one who could easily quiet down and sit in full lotus position. I kept practicing. Years later, in my early teens, I discovered by chance that I could dispel clouds and make the sun come out if I could free myself entirely of random thoughts and call sincerely in the direction of the sun. That was a key experience. It proved to me that human beings and the universe were connected, that the universal energy responded to contact. I had many questions that no textbook could answer. I became interested in Buddhist and Daoist philosophy.

When I was still in high school I went to one of the four most famous Buddhist Temples in China, to Nan Hai Pu Tuo. This is where Guanyin became enlightened. There, I was lucky to be instructed in many 'secret' practices by Abbess Huikong herself. Her teachings and those of other grand masters later convinced me that man and the universe are united, are one and the same, and I realized that this had epochal meaning for the well-being of everyone on this planet.

I studied philosophy, graduated, started teaching. But the Chinese Qigong Research Society and the Somatic Science Association invited me to give presentations and workshops. They became very successful, and a lot of healings happened. So finally I said good bye to my academic career and founded a small Qigong College—the Modern Purple Bamboo College—which I promoted on a national scale.

McLaughlin: I understand that you developed your

own Qigong system. Why? And how does it differ from traditional systems?

Qinyin: My teaching made me realize that traditional Qigong at times was too complicated, or obscure, and practice took a long time before health benefits became apparent. I also realized that people nowadays are more stressed than ever, and have less time. I wanted to design the most efficient, quickest way for healing. So I closed my college for a while and searched for legendary masters residing in the countryside, and difficult to find. I managed, after much hardship, to be instructed by some extraordinary hermits, and I explored and experimented on myself. I discovered that health benefits could be achieved quickly if qi could be used for getting rid of toxins. So I combined qi infusion with detoxification in an energized fasting of varied length for different people, and the results were astounding. I also streamlined traditional qigong practices into a set of simple clear and more powerful Qigong exercises.

These innovations in theory and practice I offer under Qin-Way to Health and Rejuvenation in an energized fasting workshop and subsequent advanced workshops that build on the completion of this first one, and ultimately teach the trainee to become a healer. In the workshop participants learn to open up their acupuncture points and energy channels and connect with universal energy almost immediately. The attendants were able to fill themselves with qi-instead of food, expel toxins, and miraculously heal hypertension, diabetes, overweight, arthritis, skin diseases, insomnia, migraine, and other chronic ailments.

McLaughlin: How would you say qigong differs from other practices such as Taiji, Yoga, or Zen Meditation?

Qinyin: Taiji shares with Qigong that it also aims at the maintenance of health and at healing, but Taiji includes the study of self-defense, of developing martial arts power, which Qi-Gong does not. Both coordinate breath and movements, and fine-tune awareness of the different kinds of breathing and the states of consciousness breathing awakens.

Again, there are lots of parallels between Qigong and Yoga which originated in India. Yoga is also about accumulating prana, life energy, through breath control exercises and physical postures. It also has a yin-yang theory of balancing solar and lunar currents of life energy, and it is probably older than qigong and may have influenced its development. Movements in Qi Gong tend to be circular and slow; and holding stances are less frequent than in Yoga postures. In Qi Gong, often long sequences of movements are taught, but not in my system. Zen meditation tries to achieve the point of inner stillness and balance through meditation alone, and considers this the precondition for health and healing.

Anyway, there are many different versions of Qigong. A major characteristic of Qinway Qigong is that it opens the energy channels between the human being and the universe in a short time and accumulates energy slowly.

McLaughlin: What do you mean by detoxification?

Qinyin: It operates on the physical and mental level. You get rid of toxins and metabolic wastes in your physical body. And, just as important, you let go of incorrect or harmful information, and you aim at being spiritually pure. That is, you aim at cultivating positive emotions—equanimity, kindness, compassion, patience, love, happiness, for example, and you want to repent and avoid such negative feelings as anger, hatred, jealousy, envy, impatience, greed, self-righteousness etc. which are the toxins of your mind or soul and undermine your health. In other words, the goal is to find the balance point between yin and yang, a place of stillness in the midst of movement. (like Thoreau's witness self, I think to myself)

McLaughlin: Given that we are overstressed and eager to get quick results with as little effort as possible, is there something you recommend that will have an immediate positive effect on our health?

Qinyin: Yes, the best is really my energized fasting and detoxification retreat. I give them regularly at my home in Fremont, and soon, Sept. 15-17, this year at the Land of the Medicine Buddha. I connect people with universal energy; give them a tape with exercise directions and music, energized for them; and twice daily I send them energy, they drink energized tea and water, and eat an energized date.

McLaughlin: How long do people fast and how do they feel?

Qinyin: The longest fast was over forty days, and a rare skin disease disappeared and the person lost many pounds permanently. People feel differently, depending on what kind and how many toxins they have in their bodies. It is common to feel cold, or hot, tired, weak, you may perspire and urinate more; you probably will discharge tarry stool, you might smell badly, get a rash, maybe vomit. And a lot of people feel very few symptoms. They are usually not hungry. The minimum fast is three days, and the average people fast is a week to ten days.

McLaughlin: Where do you think Qi Gong will take me as I go deeper into its practice?

Qinyin: That's hard to predict. You will probably eat less, feel more energized and lighter, you will probably shift your diet and eat fewer acidifying foods, such as meats and grains, and more alkalizing foods such as vegetables and fruits. You will become more sensitive and gentle, feel more loving and kind toward yourself and others, more emotionally balanced and joyful. You might sense the energy in other people, in foods, in pictures, in things and beings around you. That is, you will stay in a qi-field most of the time. You are not likely to get ill a lot. You might communicate with universal energy, and have it support your wishes.

McLaughlin (jokingly): Do you think I'll be able to bend a steel spoon as you did with such ease a while ago?

Qinyin (laughing): Who knows, you might! It means that you have to be able to accumulate a tremendous amount of qi inside and then direct it at will.

McLaughlin: What's your reaction to the political turmoil surrounding Qigong in China?

Qinyin: I think the turmoil surrounding Qigong in China is not surprising. It is very easy for a version of Qigong to become a political factor, if it has many followers and behaves in a special way. Qigong sometimes brings about supernatural phenomena. It is not surprising this may conflict with current official science and politics.

McLaughlin: what are your plans for the future here in the United States?

Qinyin: I would like to have an institute for teaching my qigong, for training other teachers, and also for healing people who can't get help anywhere else at low cost. In fact, I am looking for a foundation or a person who would provide me some seed money for the project. I am very eager to share my knowledge and benefit others with it.

CHAPTER 18

Fasting for Self-Cleansing

To undertake fasting for self-cleansing, it is essential to drop all expectations and all information that we have read or heard because it will only interfere with our inner process, which is unique to us only. The real work is unseen and it may not be felt or recognized for months. Usually what happens is the exact opposite of what is expected or demanded in a fixed way, according to experts.

Why Fasting ?

Fasting is an essential ingredient of most spiritual practices since ancient times (Jesus, Moses, Mohammed, Buddha etc.) and is based on the recognition of the body as the "temple of our consciousness."

The body needs to be adequately prepared to sustain different levels of spiritual experiences. Dense matter and lower vibrations need to be traded off with light/prana so that we can evolve.

Fasting is a form of healing and its main focal point is that when eating is stopped the body shifts into a state of detoxification. Cells start releasing unwanted toxic material into the bloodstream with the intention to eliminate it via the elimination organs—colon, liver, kidneys, lungs, skin and the lymphatic system.

Fasting goes gradually into deeper layers of detoxification. The first cycle is skipping a single meal. "Hunger" occurs after 4 hours, 9 hours, 18 hours, 36 hours, $3\frac{1}{4}$ days, 1 week, 2 weeks, 3 weeks, 6 weeks and so on.

The feeling of hunger is emotionally rather than physically based because we can always intentionally bypass it. Long-term fasters, liquidarians, breatharians are living proof of this.

A critical point is the 36 hours after which the actual cellular detoxification is activated and the lymphatic system starts moving substantial quantities of toxins.

In one week the entire bloodstream has been cleansed to the degree that a person's consciousness has allowed no more or less of what has been appropriate for the time being.

Why Cleansing ?

The essence of the cleansing program is to recognize how our choices affect our being and choose consciously to take the responsibility for these choices. The purpose is not to get rid of toxicity.

This is denial of a part of ourselves and it cannot be exorcised. It will keep coming back until we feel at peace with all the parts of our psyche.

The purpose is to recognize the parts of ourselves that have served us in the past (so we can evolve where we are now) and now we choose to move onto a lighter sphere of existence.

The fact that these parts are no longer serving our current needs doesn't mean that we act irresponsibly, denying that we have needed them in the past and denying them as alien beings.

They are part of our consciousness and they need to be accepted, appreciated, respected and loved, not rejected and denied. Our sincere gratitude is the only key to their graceful evaporation and transmutation into light.

In fact, the "toxic" energy accumulated inside of us

doesn't go away, it simply transmutes into a lighter form more useful to our current needs and choices.

The toxicity accumulated and any physical or emotional imbalances are simply our choices. We (our consciousness at a deep level) chose it when our mind failed to perceive the natural harmony on a subtle level.

Then we simply project it in a more dense vibration so our physical body can respond and recognize the imbalance.

Even when our mind ignored these signs, our consciousness still kept persisting to heal the imbalance by "knocking at the door stronger." We simply need to pay attention to these signs.

There is no need to react because there is no threat. It is the consciousness attempting to heal our wounds and simply ask for our conscious cooperation.

It may sound funny, but we need to love our shit, recognizing that Consciousness out of wisdom and love, encapsulated all dense energy in mucus and has deposited it safely in parts of the body, gracefully and patiently.

It has tolerated years of abuse, ignorance, arrogance and disrespect of the Natural Laws, until we are ready to recognize it and reverse the process.

We may either choose to deny any involvement/ responsibility, or choose to express our gratitude for all this love that serves us by protecting our physical body each moment we are alive.

What is really doing all the work ?

The real cleansing work is done by consciousness-our inner healing mechanism. The supplements, herbs, water etc. are simply to provide the necessary nurturing and support to the organs and bodily systems that go through a very intense detox experience.

After a number of fasts and cleanses there is no need for any supplement because the body recognizes the intention and becomes entrained and very efficient in detoxifying itself.

Even toxic food doesn't hurt the body if it is taken occasionally, consciously, responsibly and without denial, ignorance or arrogance. It is a process of trust and surrender to our inner wisdom.

It penetrates all levels of our being, most importantly our cellular system, and transfers vital consciousness information that registers in the cells. It becomes a point of reference from now onwards, pulling magnetically the body-mind to a higher vibrational frequency.

This is what is really happening. The fasting—cleansing process accelerates healing towards a higher vibrational state of existence.

It has been observed, over a period of years, that fasting people release less dense material, but they are also transformed much deeper. Probably this reflects the raising of the vibrational frequency of the planet and the increased number of beings resonating to this raising!

Healing Crisis

Don't forget that cleansing reactions do not last (unless we keep stubbornly resisting), and they indicate that a healing crisis is at work. Healing crises are the body's natural Detoxification mechanism. They bring to the surface and flush out the original cause of the imbalance (or the appropriate layer at that time.)

Healing crises are the wisest guides we could ever have and are only offered to people who have earned it through their strong intention or commitment (even unconsciously.)

Healing crises are always chosen and invited by our deepest self, and therefore can never hurt us. We'll never invite something unnecessary or something we are unable to handle at the time. Our welcoming of the healing, or our resistance, holds the key in how we experience each healing crisis.

There can be no health restoration without some sort of healing crisis sooner or later. It feels exactly like an infected wound. If we decide to heal it by disinfecting it, it would probably hurt for a while but it is obviously the only way.

However, when a Healing Crisis persists it becomes obvious that (unless we decide to let go of the associated blockage) we may not be ready for the release and we shouldn't stubbornly torture ourselves. We can do it later on, when we are ready.

Feeling "Weakness" and "No Energy"

More people nowadays are feeling increasingly "weak" and "tired" during the fast, as compared to a few years ago. Yet this is actually an illusion of the mind. Fasting allows much more energy to be utilized, but is mostly directed into the healing of what is essential and not to entertain our mind's familiar patterns.

It is a period of time when not only does our mind need to be more still, but also our body needs to be still. We don't need to be "energetic," or "feel good." It is entirely irrelevant to the healing process. If we listen to our consciousness by observing the body signs, we'll quickly recognize that we need to listen and pay attention to subtle shifts. This requires physical stillness. We need to remember that.

Digesting Emotions and Beliefs

Sometimes we may wonder why we have digestive/ assimilation/elimination problems, even though our eating habits are relatively or remarkably healthy.

We may need to consider that the vibration of our emotional choices and mental attitudes (Anger, Fear, Mistrust, etc.) form dense vibrations that become part of our being and interfere with the free flow of life. It is not simply the food we ingest. It is also emotions and beliefs.

An Interesting Nutritional—Diet Suggestion

Let's choose any nutritional system that we feel comfortable with: combination diet, raw food diet, Chinese, fish and chicken, macrobiotic, lacto vegetarian, vegan, fruitarian, breatharian.

Then, identify our choice as our main diet for any time period i.e. 2 weeks or 2 months, etc.

Anytime during that period any cravings for "prohibited foods, drinks etc." WE DO NOT SUPPRESS and DO NOT FEEL GUILTY ABOUT. We can simply write them down and allow ourselves to enjoy all of them in 1-2 days with no barriers and no remorse.

We can treat and reward the part of us that craves. We can acknowledge it and satisfy its needs but only during that predetermined time period. After that "junk food day" we can do a good cleanse of e.g. a weekend fast on juices and water with perhaps enemas/colonics, if possible, and psyllium support if possible.

Then we can go back to our chosen diet. In this simple way there is no suppression, no guilt, no abuse. We bring consciousness into all modes: our healthy eating, our emotional enjoyment, and our fasting-cleansing.

Our Consciousness honours our body and therefore there is no toxicity endangerment.

We enjoy all choices and we feel empowered to choose our desired state rather than feeling enslaved constantly satisfying cravings or being trapped in a rigid healthy diet.

Acknowledge, appreciate and love the whole of ourselves.

CHAPTER 19

Prana and Your Third Eye

Osho Rajneesh narrates how when Pythagoras reached Egypt to enter a school, a secret esoteric school of mysticism, he was refused admission. And Pythagoras was one of the best minds ever produced. He could not understand it. He applied again and again, but he was told that unless he goes through a particular training of fasting and breathing he couldn't be allowed to enter the school.

Pythagoras is reported to have said, "I have come for knowledge, not for any sort of discipline." But the school authorities said, "We cannot give you knowledge unless you are different and, really, we are not interested in knowledge at all. We are interested in actual experience. And no knowledge is knowledge unless it is lived and experienced. So you will have to go on a forty-day fast, continuously breathing in a certain manner, with a certain awareness on certain points." There was no other way, so Pythagoras had to pass through this training. After forty days of fasting and breathing, aware, attentive, he was allowed to enter the school. It is said that Pythagoras said, "You are not allowing Pythagoras. I am a different man. I am reborn. And you were right and I was wrong. My whole standpoint was intellectual. Through this purification my center of being has changed. From the intellect it has come down to the heart. Now I can feel things. Before this training I could

only understand through the intellect, through the head.
Now I can feel. Now Truth is not a concept to me, but a
life. It is not going to be a philosophy, but, rather, an
experience — existential."

What was that training he went through?

This fifth technique was that technique that was given
to Pythagoras. It was given in Egypt, but that technique is
very, very old.

The technique: "Attention between eyebrows, let mind
be before thought. Let form fill with breath essence the
top of the head and then a shower of light."

This was the technique given to Pythagoras.
Pythagoras went with this technique to Greece. And,
really, he became the fountainhead, the source, of all
mysticism in the West. He is the father of all gnosticism
in the West. He was the real originator of sacred
geometry. He developed it as fun game for exploration
of divine influence on the earth. Leonardo da Vinci was
introduced to this technique and became one of the
leaders of the order. Isaac Newton was also one of the
initiates and leaders. His alchemical works connected to
this technique was preparation to his gravitation theory.
Niels Bohr used it for development of what we know
today as quantum physics. In his book "What is life?"
Mr. Shrodinger, Nobel prize winner, gave one of the best
foundations for DNA understanding.

This technique is one of the very deep methods. Try to
understand this: "Attention between the eyebrows..."
Modern physiology, scientific research says that between
the two eyebrows is the gland which is a very mysterious
part in the body. This gland, called the pineal gland, is
the third eye of the Tibetans—"Shivanetra", the eye of
Shiva in the tantra. Between the two eyes there is a third
eye existing, but it is non-functioning. It is there; it can
function any moment. But it is not functioning
naturally. You have to do something about it to open it.

It is not blind. It is simply closed. This technique is to open the third eye.

"Attention between the eyebrows..."

Close your eyes, then focus both of your eyes just in the middle of the two eyebrows. Focus just in the: middle, with closed eyes, as if you are looking with your two eyes. Give total attention to it.

This is one of the simplest methods of being attentive. You cannot be attentive to any other part of the body so easily. This gland absorbs attention unlike anything else. If you give attention to it, your both eyes become hypnotized with the third eye. They become fixed; they cannot move. If you are trying to be attentive to any other part of the body it is difficult. This third eye catches attention, forces attention. It is magnet for attention. So all the methods all over the world have used it. It is the simplest to train attention because not only are you trying to be attentive: the gland itself helps you; it is magnetic. Your attention is brought to it forcibly. It is absorbed. It is said in the old tantra scriptures that for the third eye attention is food. It is hungry; it has been hungry forever. If you pay attention to it, it becomes alive. It becomes alive! The food is given to it. And once you know that attention is food, only you feel that your attention is magnetically drawn, attracted, pulled by the gland itself, attention is not a difficult thing then. One needs only to know the right point. So just close your eyes, let your two eyes move just in the middle, and feel the point. When you are near the point, suddenly your eyes will become fixed. When it will be difficult to move them, then know you have caught the right point.

"Attention between the eyebrows. Let mind be before thought..." If this attention is there, for the first time you will come to experience a strange phenomenon. For the first time you will feel thoughts running before you; you will become the witness. It is just like a film screen:

thoughts are running and you are a witness. Once your attention is focused at the third eye center, you become immediately the witness of thoughts. Ordinarily you are not the witness: you are identified with thoughts. If anger is there, you become anger. If a thought moves, you are not the witness: you become one with the thought-identified and you move with it. You become the thought; you take the form of the thought. When sex is there you become sex, when anger is there you become anger, when greed is there you become greed. Any thought moving becomes identified with you. You do not have any gap between you and the thought. In this state of mind you never know Who You Are. You are only projection of your thoughts. You can not stop them. You can not control them. Your real Self is something far away of you!

But focused at the third eye, suddenly you become the witness. You become you real Self. You become the real "I am". Through the third eye, you become the Awaken. Through the third eye, you can see thoughts running like clouds in the sky or like people moving on the street. When you are sitting at your window looking at the sky or at people in the street: you are not identified. You are peaceful and mindful, a watcher on the hill; centered in Self. Now if anger is there, you can look at it as an object.

Now you do not feel that YOU are angry. You feel that you are surrounded by anger: a cloud of anger has come around you. But you are not the anger—and if you are not that anger, anger becomes impotent. It cannot affect you; you remain untouched. The anger will come and go, and you will remain centered in yourself and your peace.

This technique is a technique of finding of the I am Presence. "Attention between the eyebrows, let the mind be before thought": now look at your thoughts;

now encounter your thoughts. "Let form fill with breath essence to the top of the head and there, shower of light": When attention is focused at the third-eye center, between the two eyebrows, two things happen. One, suddenly you become a witness. This can happen in two ways. You become a witness, and you will be centered at the third eye.

Try to be a witness. Whatsoever is happening, try to be a witness. You are ill, the body is aching and painful, you leave misery and suffering, whatsoever: be a witness to it. Whatsoever is happening, do not identify yourself with it. Be the "I am Presence"—an observer. Then if I am Presence becomes possible, you will be focused in the third eye.

Secondly, vice versa is the case also. If you are focused in the third eye, you will become a I am Presence. These two things are part of one. So try first thing: by being centered in the third eye there will be the arising of the Self. Now you can encounter your thoughts. This will be the first thing. And the second thing will be that now you can feel the subtle, delicate vibration of all energies in your body. Now you can feel the vibrations, waveforms and energy of breathing, that deep essence of breathing.

First try to understand what is meant by "Let: form" by "the essence of breathing". While you are breathing, you are not only breathing air. Science says you are breathing only air—just oxygen, hydrogen, and other gasses in there combined form of air. They say you are breathing "air"! But tantra says that air is just the vehicle, not the real thing. You are breathing "prana"— vitality. Air is just the medium; prana is the content. You are breathing prana—not only air.

Modern science is still not able to find out whether there is something like prana. But some researchers have felt something mysterious. Breathing is not simply air.

Many modern researchers have felt it also. In particular, one name is to be mentioned. Wilhelm Reich, a German psychologist who called it "orgone energy". It is the same thing as prana. He says that while you are breathing, air is just the container, and there is a mysterious content, which can be, called "orgon" or "prana" or "elan vital". But that is very subtle. Really, it is not material. Air is the material thing: the container is material. But something subtle, non-material, is moving through it.

Reich explored in detail influence of this energy to emotional life. He found that people with distracted energy flow have emotional and sexual difficulties. He developed various breathing and body exercises to facilitate free flow and prana absorption. He realized, a thing well known to tantrics, that if you give yourself free flow and sufficient prana accumulation you will enter the ecstasy, cosmic orgasm and divine bliss. Therefore, he called this energy "orgasmic energy". This is the best healing method ever developed.

Wilhelm Reich did many experiments, but he was thought to be a mad man. Science has its own superstitions, and science is a very orthodox thing. Science cannot feel yet that there is any thing more than air, but India has been experimenting with it for centuries.

You may have heard or you have even seen someone going into Samadhi (Cosmic Consciousness)—underground Samadhi for days together, with no air penetrating. One man went into such underground Samadhi in Egypt, in 1880, for forty years. Those who had buried him all died, because he was to come out of his Samadhi in 1920, forty years afterwards. In 1920. no one believed that they would find him alive, but he was found alive. He lived afterwards for ten years more. He had become completely pale, but he was alive. And there was no possibility of air reaching to him.

Medical doctors and others asked him, "What is the secret of it?" He said, "We do not know. We only know this, that prana can enter and flow anywhere." Air cannot penetrate, but prana can penetrate. Once you know that you can suck prana directly, without the container, then you can go into Samadhi for centuries even.

By being focused in the third eye, suddenly you can observe the real essence of breath-not breath, but the real essence of breath-prana. And if you can observe the essence of breath, prana, you are on the point from where the jump, the breakthrough, happens.

The technique says, "Let form fill with breath essence to the top of the head..." And when you come to feel the essence of breathing, prana, just imagine that your head is filled with it. Just imagine. No need of any effort. You just need to gently invoke the thought. I will explain to you how manifestation works. When you are focused at the third eye center, imagine, and the thing happens — then and there. Now your imagination is just important. You go on imagining, and nothing happens. But sometimes, unknowingly, in ordinary life also, things happen. You are imagining about your friend, and suddenly there is a ring on the phone. You say it is a coincidence that the friend has called you.

Sometimes your imagination works just like coincidence. But whenever this happens, now try and remember, and analyze the whole thing. Whenever it happens that you feel your imagination has become actual, go inside and observe.

Somewhere your attention must have been near the third eye. Whenever this coincidence happens, it is not a coincidence. It looks that way because you do not know the secret science. Your mind must have moved unknowingly near the third-eye center. If your attention is in the third eye, just gentle tough is enough to create any phenomenon.

This technique says that when you are focused between the eyebrows and you can feel the very essence of breathing. Now imagine that this essence is filling your whole head particularly the top of the head, the "Crown Chakra" (the highest psychic center). And the moment you imagine, it will be filled. "There at the top of the head, shower of light": This prana essence is showering from the top of your head as light. And it WILL begin to shower, and under the shower of light you will be refreshed, reborn, completely' new. It will start the new recharging of your dormant parts of DNA and it will start creation of your Light Body. At this moment your Third Eye will activate your Crown Chakra. Pineal gland will send the an order to Pituitary gland for production of Divine hormones. Some specific cells need to awaken in your Pituitary gland and they will start with production of Divine Hormones. There cells were active before your were born, during your life in mother womb. Then your prana and kundalini energy were flowing freely, you were most of the time in state of Cosmic Samadhi. You were able to leave the body and travel with your soul wherever you like. Have you ever seen a picture of a 5-6 month old fetus? They look like the most spiritual beings on Earth and really they are. In Vedic literature this Divine hormone is called "Soma—the man into God transforming substance". Soma will activate your dormant parts of DNA and transform you into the Immoralist with Light Body. That is what inner re-birth means.

So two things: first, focused on the third eye, your thoughts become potent, powerful. That is why so much insistence has been given to purity: before doing these practices, be pure. Purity is not a moral concept. Purity is significant because if you are focused at the third eye and your mind is impure, your imagination can become dangerous: dangerous to you, dangerous to others. If you are thinking of murdering someone, if this idea is in the mind, just imagining may kill the man. That is why so much insistence on being pure first. Pythagoras was told to go through fasting, through particular breathing — this breathing, because impure you will have a lot of difficulties to reach this point and then it could be dangerous.

You might have observed someone being hypnotized. When someone is hypnotized, the hypnotist can say anything and immediately the hypnotized person follows.

Howsoever absurd the order, howsoever irrational or even impossible, the hypnotized person follows it. What is happening? This technique. It is at the base of all hypnotism. Whenever someone is being hypnotized he is told to focus his eyes at a particular point on some light, some dot on the wall, or anything or on the eyes of the hypnotist.

When you focus your eyes at any particular point, within three minutes your inner attention begins to flow toward the third eye. At the moment your inner attention begins to flow toward the third eye, your face begins to change and the hypnotist knows when your face begins to change. Suddenly your face loses all vitality. It becomes dead, as if deeply asleep. Immediately the hypnotist knows when your face has lost the lush, the aliveness. It means that now attention is being sucked by the third-eye center. Your face has become dead; the whole energy is going toward the third-eye center.

Now the hypnotist immediately knows that anything-said will happen. He says, "Now you are falling into a deep sleep": you will fall immediately. He says, "Now you have all connecting Cosmic Conscious": you will have Cosmic Conscious immediately. Now anything can be done. If he says, "Now invoke and channel the Holy Spirit of your Guardian Angel," you will start to channel them.

You will begin to behave like a your Guardian Angel, you will begin to talk like your Guardian Angel. Your gestures will change. Your unconscious will take the order and will create the actuality. If you are suffering from a disease, now it can be ordered that the disease has disappeared, and it will disappear.

Or, any new disease can be created. Just by putting an ordinary stone from the street on your hand, the hypnotist can say, "This is fire on your hand." You will feel intense heat; your hand will get burned - not only in the mind, but actually. Actually your skin will get burned. You will have a burning sensation.

What is happening? There is no fire. There is just an ordinary stone - cold.

How? How does this burning happen. You are focused at the third-eye center, your imagination is being given suggestions by the hypnotist, and they are being actualized.

This happens because of the third eye. In the third eye, thought and manifestation are not two things. Imagination is the fad. Imagine, and it is so.

There is no gap between dream and reality. There is no gap between dream and reality I dream, and it will become real. That is why great saints has said that this whole world is nothing but the dream of the Divine— the DREAM of the Divine! This is because the Divines is centered in the third eye—always, eternally. So whatsoever the Divine dreams, it becomes real. If you are also centered in the third eye, whatsoever you dream will become real.

One day Sariputta came to Buddha. He meditated deeply, then many things, many visions, started coming, as it happens with anyone who goes into deep meditation. He began to see heavens, he began to see hells, and he began to see angels, gods, and demons. And they were actual, so real; that he came again to

Buddha to tell him that such and such a vision had come to him. But Buddha said, "It is nothing—just dreams. Just dreams" But Sariputta said, "They are so real. How can I say that they are dreams? When I see a flower in my vision it is more real than any flower in the world. The fragrance is there; I can touch it. When I see you," he said to Buddha, "it is not as real. That flower is more real than your being here just before me, so how can I differentiate what is real and what is dream ".Buddha said, "Now that you are centered in the third eye, dream and reality are one. Whatsoever you are dreaming will be real, and vice versa also." For one who is centred in the third eye, dreams will become real and the whole reality will become just a dream, because when your dream can become real, you know there is no basic difference between dream and reality. So when your guru says that this whole world is just maya, a dream of the Divine, it is not a theoretical proposition, it is not a philosophical statement. It is, rather, the inner experience of one who is focused in the third eye.

CHAPTER 20

Honouring Prana

Vedic scholar Dr. David Frawley narrates an old Vedic story about Prana that we find in various Upanishads. The five main faculties of our nature—the mind, breath (prana), speech, ear and eye—were arguing with each other as to which one of them was the best and most important. This reflects the ordinary human state in which our faculties are not integrated but fight with each other, competing for their rule over our attention. To resolve this dispute they decided that each would leave the body and see whose absence was most missed.

First speech left the body but the body continued though mute. Next the eye left but the body continued though blind. Next the ear left but the body continued though deaf. Mind left but the body continued though unconscious. Finally, the Prana began to leave and the body began to die and all the other faculties began to lose their energy. So all they all rushed to Prana and told it to stay, lauding its supremacy. Clearly, Prana won the argument. Prana gives energy to all our faculties, without which they cannot function.

Without honouring Prana first there is nothing else we can do and no energy with which to do anything. The moral of this story is that to control our faculties the key is the control of Prana.

Prana has many levels of meaning from the breath to the energy of consciousness itself. Prana is not only the

basic life-force, it is the master form of all energy working
on the level of mind, life and body. Indeed, the entire
universe is a manifestation of Prana, which is the original
creative power. Even Kundalini Shakti, the serpent
power or inner power that transforms consciousness,
develops from the awakened Prana.

On a cosmic level there are two basic aspects of Prana.
The first is the unmanifest aspect of Prana, which is the
energy of Pure Consciousness that transcends all
creation. The second or manifest Prana is the force of
creation itself. Prana arises from the quality (guna) of
rajas, the active force of Nature (Prakriti). Nature herself
consists of three gunas: sattva or harmony, which gives
rise to the mind, rajas or movement, which gives rise to
the prana, and tamas or inertia that gives rise to the body.

Indeed it could be argued that Prakriti or Nature is
primarily Prana or rajas. Nature is an active energy or
Shakti. According to the pull or attraction of the higher
Self or pure consciousness (Purusha) this energy becomes
sattvic. By the inertia of ignorance this energy becomes
tamasic.

However, even the Purusha or higher Self can be said
to be unmanifest Prana because it is a form of energy of
consciousness (Devatma Shakti or Citi Shakti). From the
unmanifest Prana of Pure Awareness comes the manifest
Prana of creation, through which the entire universe
comes into being.

Relative to our physical existence, Prana or vital energy
is a modification of the air element, primarily the oxygen
we breathe that allows us to live. Yet as air originates in
ether or space, Prana arises in space and remains closely
connected to it. Wherever we create space there energy
or Prana must arise automatically.

The element of air relates to the sense of touch in the
Yogic system. Air on a subtle level is touch. Through
touch we feel alive and can transmit our life-force to

others. Yet as air arises in space, so does touch arises from sound, which is the sense quality that corresponds to the element of ether. Through sound we awaken and feel our broader connections with life as a whole. On a subtle level Prana arises from the touch and sound qualities that are inherent in consciousness. In fact, Prana has its own sheath or body.

The human being consists of five koshas or sheaths:

1. *Annamaya kosha:* food—physical—the five elements;
2. *Pranamaya kosha:* breath—vital—the five pranas;
3. *Manomaya kosha:* impressions—outer mind—the five kinds of sensory impressions;
4. *Vijnanamaya kosha:* ideas - intelligence—directed mental activity; and
5. *Anandamaya kosha:* experiences—deeper mind— memory, subliminal and superconscious mind.

Pranamaya Kosha

The Pranamaya Kosha is the sphere of our vital life energies. This sheath mediates between the body on one side and the three sheaths of the mind (outer mind, intelligence and inner mind) on the other and has an action on both levels. It meditates between the five gross elements and the five sensory impressions.

The best English term for the Pranamaya kosha is probably the "vital sheath" or "vital body," to use a term from Sri Aurobindo's Integral Yoga. Pranamaya kosha consists of our vital urges of survival, reproduction, movement and self-expression, being mainly connected to the five motor organs (excretory, urino-genital, feet, hands, and vocal organ).

Most of us are dominated by the vital body and its deep-seated urges that are necessary for us to remain alive. It is also the home of the vital or subconscious ego which holds the various fears, desires and attachments which afflict us. We most of our spend our time in life seeking enjoyment through the vital in the form of sensory enjoyment and acquisition of material objects.

A person with a strong vital nature becomes prominent in life and is able to impress his personality upon the world. Those with a weak vital lack the power to accomplish much of anything and have little effect upon life, usually remaining in a subordinate position. Generally people with strong and egoistic vitals run the world, while those with weak vitals follow them. Such a strong egoistic vital is one of the greatest obstacles to the spiritual path.

A strong vital or Pranamaya kosha, however, is important for the spiritual path as well, but this is very different than the egoistic or desire oriented vital. It derives its strength not from our personal power but from surrender to the Divine and its great energy. Without a strong spiritual vital we lack the power to do our practices and not fall under worldly influences. In Hindu mythology this higher Prana is symbolized by the monkey God Hanuman, the son of the Wind, who surrendered to the Divine in the form of Sita-Rama, can become as large or small as he wishes, can overcome all enemies and obstacles, and accomplish the miraculous. Such a spiritual vital has energy, curiosity and enthusiasm in life along with a control of the senses and vital urges, with their subordination to a higher will and aspiration.

Pranamaya kosha is composed of the five Pranas. The one primary Prana divides into five types according to its movement and direction. This is an important subject in Ayurvedic medicine as well as Yogic thought.

Prana

Prana, literally the "forward moving air," moves inward and governs reception of all types from the eating of food, drinking of water, and inhalation of air, to the reception of sensory impressions and mental experiences. It is propulsive in nature, setting things in motion and guiding them. It provides the basic energy that drives us in life.

Apana

Apana, literally the "air that moves away," moves downward and outward and governs all forms of elimination and reproduction (which also has a downward movement). It governs the elimination of the stool and the urine, the expelling of semen, menstrual fluid and the fetus, and the elimination of carbon dioxide through the breath. On a deeper level it rules the elimination of negative sensory, emotional and mental experiences. It is the basis of our immune function on all levels.

Udana

Udana, literally the "upward moving air," moves upward and qualitative or transformative movements of the life-energy. It governs growth of the body, the ability to stand, speech, effort, enthusiasm and will. It is our main positive energy in life through which we can develop our different bodies and evolve in consciousness.

Samana

Samana, literally the "balancing air," moves from the periphery to the center, through a churning and discerning action. It aids in digestion on all levels. It works in the gastrointestinal tract to digest food, in the lungs to digest air or absorb oxygen, and in the mind to homogenize and digest experiences, whether sensory, emotional or mental.

Vyana

Vyana, literally the "outward moving air," moves from the center to the periphery. It governs circulation on all levels. It moves the food, water and oxygen throughout the body, and keeps our emotions and thoughts circulating in the mind, imparting movement and providing strength. In doing so it assists all the other Pranas in their work.

The five Pranas are energies and processes that occur on several levels. However we can localize them in a few key ways. Prana Vayu governs the movement of energy from the head down to the navel, which is the Pranic center in the physical body. Apana Vayu governs the movement of energy from the navel down to the root chakra. Samana Vayu governs the movement of energy from the entire body back to the navel. Vyana Vayu governs the movement of energy out from the navel throughout the entire body. Udana governs the movement of energy from the navel up to the head As a simple summary we could say that Prana governs the intake of substances. Samana governs their digestion. Vyana governs the circulation of nutrients. Udana governs the release of positive energy. Apana governs the elimination of waste-materials.

This is much like the working of a machine. Prana brings in the fuel, Samana converts this fuel to energy, Vyana circulates the energy to the various work sites. Apana releases the waste materials or by products of the conversion process. Udana governs the positive energy created in the process and determines the work that the machine is able to do.

The key to health and well-being is to keep our Pranas in harmony. When one Prana becomes imbalanced, the others tend to become imbalanced as well because they are all linked together. Generally Prana and Udana work opposite to Apana as the forces of energization versus those of elimination. Similarly, Vyana and Samana are opposites as expansion and contraction.

Yoga is a vast system of spiritual practices for inner

growth. To this end, the classical yoga system incorporates eight limbs, each with its own place and function. Of these, pratyahara is probably the least known. How many people, even yoga teachers, can define pratyahara? Have you ever taken a class in pratyahara? Have you ever seen a book on pratyahara? Can you think of several important pratyahara techniques? Do you perform pratyahara as part of your yogic practices? Yet unless we understand pratyahara, we are missing an integral aspect of yoga without which the system cannot work.

As the fifth of the eight limbs, pratyahara occupies a central place. Some yogis include it among the outer aspects of yoga, others with the inner aspects. Both classifications are correct, for pratyahara is the key between the outer and inner aspects of yoga; it shows us how to move from one to the other.

It is not possible to move directly from asana to meditation. This requires jumping from the body to the mind, forgetting what lies between. To make this transition, the breath and senses, which link the body and mind, must be brought under control and developed properly. This is where pranayama and pratyahara come in. With pranayama we control our vital energies and impulses and with pratyahara we gain mastery over the unruly senses—both prerequisites to successful meditation.

What is Pratyahara?

The term pratyahara is composed of two Sanskrit words, prati and ahara. Ahara means "food," or "anything we take into ourselves from the outside." Prati is a preposition meaning "against" or "away." Pratyahara means literally "control of ahara," or "gaining mastery over external influences." It is compared to a turtle withdrawing its limbs into its shell — the turtle's shell is the mind and the senses are the limbs. The term is usually translated as "withdrawal from the senses," but much more is implied.

In yogic thought there are three levels of ahara, or food. The first is physical food that brings in the five elements necessary to nourish the body. The second is impressions, which bring in the subtle substances necessary to nourish the mind — the sensations of sound, touch, sight, taste, and smell. The third level of ahara is our associations, the people we hold at heart level who serve to nourish the soul and affect us with the gunas of sattva, rajas, and tamas.

Pratyahara is twofold. It involves withdrawal from wrong food, wrong impressions and wrong associations, while simultaneously opening up to right food, right impressions and right associations. We cannot control our mental impressions without right diet and right relationship, but pratyahara's primary importance lies in control of sensory impressions which frees the mind to move within.

By withdrawing our awareness from negative impressions, pratyahara strengthens the mind's powers of immunity. Just as a healthy body can resist toxins and pathogens, a healthy mind can ward off the negative sensory influences around it. If you are easily disturbed by the noise and turmoil of the environment around you, practice pratyahara. Without it, you will not be able to meditate.

There are four main forms of pratyahara: indriya-pratyahara—control of the senses; prana- pratyahara—control of prana; karma-pratyahara—control of action; and mano-pratyahara—withdrawal of mind from the senses. Each has its special methods.

1. Control of the Senses (Indriya-pratyahara): Indriya-pratyahara, or control of the senses, is the most important form of pratyahara, although this is not something that we like to hear about in our mass media-oriented culture. Most of us suffer from sensory overload, the result of constant bombardment from television, radio, computers, newspapers, magazines, books—you name it. Our commercial society functions by stimulating our interest through the senses. We are constantly confronted with bright colors, loud noises and dramatic sensations. We have been raised on every sort of sensory indulgence; it is the main form of entertainment in our society.

The problem is that the senses, like untrained children, have their own will, which is largely instinctual in nature. They tell the mind what to do. If we don't discipline them, they dominate us with their endless demands. We are so accustomed to ongoing sensory activity that we don't know how to keep our minds quiet; we have become hostages of the world of the senses and its allurements.

We run after what is appealing to the senses and forget the higher goals of life. For this reason, pratyahara is probably the most important limb of yoga for people today.

The old saying "the spirit is willing but the flesh is weak" applies to those of us who have not learned how to properly control our senses.

Indriya-pratyahara gives us the tools to strengthen the spirit and reduce its dependency on the body. Such control is not suppression (which causes eventual revolt), but proper coordination and motivation.

Right Intake of Impressions

Pratyahara centers on the right intake of impressions. Most of us are careful about the food we eat and the company we keep, but we may not exercise the same discrimination about the impressions we take in from the senses. We accept impressions via the mass media that we would never allow in our personal lives.

We let people into our houses through television and movies that we would never allow into our homes in real life! What kind of impressions do we take in every day? Can we expect that they will not have an effect on us? Strong sensations dull the mind, and a dull mind makes us act in ways that are insensitive, careless, or even violent.

According to Ayurveda, sensory impressions are the main food for the mind. The background of our mental field consists of our predominant sensory impressions.

We see this when our mind reverts to the impressions of the last song we heard or the last movie we saw. Just as junk food makes the body toxic, junk impressions make the mind toxic. Junk food requires a lot of salt, sugar, or spices to make it palatable because it is largely dead food; similarly junk impressions require powerful dramatic impressions—sex and violence—to make us feel that they are real, because they are actually just colors projected on a screen.

We cannot ignore the role sensory impressions play in making us who we are, for they build up the subconscious and strengthen the tendencies latent within it.

Trying to meditate without controlling our impressions pits our subconscious against us and prevents the development of inner peace and clarity.

Sensory Withdrawal

Fortunately we are not helpless before the barrage of sensory impressions. Pratyahara provides us many tools for managing them properly. Perhaps the simplest way to control our impressions is simply to cut them off, to spend some time apart from all sensory inputs. Just as the body benefits by fasting from food, so the mind benefits by fasting from impressions. This can be as simple as sitting to meditate with our eyes closed or taking a retreat somewhere free from the normal sensory bombardments, like at a mountain cabin. Also a "media fast," abstaining from television, radio, etc. can be a good practice to cleanse and rejuvenate the mind.

Yoni mudra is one of the most important pratyahara techniques for closing the senses. It involves using the fingers to block the sensory openings in the head—the eyes, ears, nostrils, and mouth—and allowing the attention and energy to move within. It is done for short periods of time when our prana is energized, such as immediately after practicing pranayama. (Naturally we should avoid closing the mouth and nose to the point at which we starve ourselves of oxygen.)

Another method of sense withdrawal is to keep our sense organs open but withdraw our attention from them. In this way we cease taking in impressions without actually closing off our sense organs. The most common method, shambhavi mudra, consists of sitting with the eyes open while directing the attention within, a technique used in several Buddhist systems of meditation as well. This redirection of the senses inward can be done with the other senses as well, particularly with the sense of hearing. It helps us control our mind even when the senses are functioning, as they are during the normal course of the day.

Focusing on Uniform Impressions

Another way to cleanse the mind and control the senses is to put our attention on a source of uniform impressions, such as gazing at the ocean or the blue sky.

Just as the digestive system gets short-circuited by irregular eating habits and contrary food qualities, our ability to digest impressions can be deranged by jarring or excessive impressions. And just as improving our digestion may require going on a mono-diet, like the ayurvedic use of rice and mung beans *(kicharee)*, so our mental digestion may require a diet of natural but homogeneous impressions. This technique is often helpful after a period of fasting from impressions.

Creating Positive Impressions

Another means of controlling the senses is to create positive, natural impressions. There are a number of ways to do this: meditating upon aspects of nature such as trees, flowers, or rocks, as well as visiting temples or other places of pilgrimage which are repositories of positive impressions and thoughts. Positive impressions can also be created by using incense, flowers, ghee lamps, altars, statues, and other artifacts of devotional worship.

Creating Inner Impressions

Another sensory withdrawal technique is to focus the mind on inner impressions, thus removing attention from external impressions. We can create our own inner impressions through the imagination or we can contact the subtle senses that come into play when the physical senses are quiet.

Visualization is the simplest means of creating inner impressions. In fact, most yogic meditation practices begin with some type of visualization, such as "seeing" a deity, a guru, or a beautiful setting in nature. More elaborate visualizations involve imagining deities and their worlds, or mentally performing rituals, such as offering imaginary flowers or gems to imagined deities. The artist absorbed in an inner landscape or the musician creating music are also performing inner visualizations. These are all forms of pratyahara because they clear the mental field of external impressions and create a positive inner impression to serve as the foundation of meditation.

Preliminary visualizations are helpful for most forms of meditation and can be integrated into other spiritual practices as well.

Laya Yoga is the yoga of the inner sound and light current, in which we focus on subtle senses to withdraw us from the gross senses. This withdrawal into inner sound and light is a means of transforming the mind and is another form of indriya-pratyahara.

2. Control of the Prana (Prana-Pratyahara): Control of the senses requires the development and control of prana because the senses follow prana (our vital energy). Unless our prana is strong we will not have the power to control the senses. If our prana is scattered or disturbed, our senses will also be scattered and disturbed.

Pranayama is a preparation for pratyahara. Prana is gathered in pranayama and withdrawn in pratyahara. Yogic texts describe methods of withdrawing prana from different parts of the body, starting with the toes and ending wherever we wish to fix our attention—the top of the head, the third eye, the heart or one of the other chakras.

Perhaps the best method of prana-pratyahara is to visualize the death process, in which the prana, or the life-force, withdraws from the body, shutting off all the senses from the feet to the head. Ramana Maharshi achieved Self-realization by doing this when he was a mere boy of seventeen. Before inquiring into the Self, he visualized his body as dead, withdrawing his prana into the mind and the mind into the heart. Without such complete and intense pratyahara, his meditative process would not have been successful.

3. Control of Action (Karma-Pratyahara): We cannot control the sense organs without also controlling the motor organs. In fact the motor organs involve us directly in the external world. The impulses coming in through the senses get expressed through the motor organs and this drives us to further sensory involvement. Because desire is endless, happiness consists not in getting what we want, but in no longer needing anything from the external world.

Just as the right intake of impressions gives control of the sense organs, right work and right action gives control of the motor organs. This involves karma yoga—performing selfless service and making our life a sacred ritual.

Karma-pratyahara can be performed by surrendering any thought of personal rewards for what we do, doing everything as service to God or to humanity. The Bhagavad Gita says, "Your duty is to act, not to seek a reward for what you do."

This is one kind of pratyahara. It also includes the practice of austerities that lead to control of the motor organs. For example, asana can be used to control the hands and feet, control which is needed when we sit quietly for extended periods of time.

4. Withdrawal of the Mind (Mano-Pratyahara): The yogis tell us that mind is the sixth sense organ and that it is responsible for coordinating all the other sense organs. We take in sensory impressions only where we place our mind's attention. In a way we are always practicing pratyahara. The mind's attention is limited and we give attention to one sensory impression by withdrawing the mind from other impressions. Wherever we place our attention, we naturally overlook other things.

We control our senses by withdrawing our mind's attention from them. According to the Yoga Sutras II.54: "When the senses do not conform with their own objects but imitate the nature of the mind, that is pratyahara." More specifically, it is mano-pratyahara—withdrawing the senses from their objects and directing them inward to the nature of the mind, which is formless. Vyasa's commentary on the Yoga Sutra notes that the mind is like the queen bee and the senses are the worker bees. Wherever the queen bee goes, all the other bees must follow. Thus mano-pratyahara is less about controlling the senses than about controlling the mind, for when the mind is controlled, the senses are automatically controlled.

We can practice mano-pratyahara by consciously withdrawing our attention from unwholesome impressions whenever they arise. This is the highest form of pratyahara and the most difficult; if we have not gained proficiency in controlling the senses, motor organs, and pranas, it is unlikely to work. Like wild animals, prana and the senses can easily overcome a weak mind, so it is usually better to start first with more practical methods of pratyahara.

Pratyahara and the other Limbs of Yoga: Pratyahara is related to all the limbs of yoga. All of the other limbs—from asana to samadhi—contain aspects of pratyahara. For example, in the sitting poses, which are the most important aspect of asana, both the sensory and motor organs are controlled. Pranayama contains an element of pratyahara as we draw our attention inward through the breath. Yama and niyama contain various principles and practices, like non-violence and contentment, that help us control the senses. In other words, pratyahara provides the foundation for the higher practices of yoga and is the basis for meditation. It follows pranayama (or control of prana) and, by linking prana with the mind, takes it out of the sphere of the body. Pratyahara is also linked with dharana. In pratyahara we withdraw our attention from ordinary distractions. In dharana we consciously focus that attention on a particular object, such as a mantra. Pratyahara is the negative and dharana the positive aspect of the same basic function.

Many of us find that even after years of meditation practice we have not achieved all that we expected. Trying to practice meditation without some degree of pratyahara is like trying to gather water in a leaky vessel. No matter how much water we bring in, it flows out at the same rate. The senses are like holes in the vessel of the mind. Unless they are sealed, the mind cannot hold the nectar of truth. Anyone whose periods of meditation alternate with periods of sensory indulgence is in need of pratyahara.

Pratyahara offers many methods of preparing the mind for meditation. It also helps us avoid environmental disturbances that are the source of psychological pain. Pratyahara is a marvelous tool for taking control of our lives and opening up to our inner being. It is no wonder some great yogis have called it "the most important limb of yoga." We should all remember to include it in our practice.

CHAPTER 21

Pranic Healing

Two basic principles govern pranic healing, the cleansing and energising of the patient's bioplasmic body with prana or ki. By cleansing or removing the diseased bioplasmic matter from the affected chakra and the diseased organ, and secondly by energising these affected parts with sufficient prana or ki, healing is achieved.

There are seven basic techniques followed in the practice of elementary pranic healing according to Choa Kok Sui: (1) Sensitising the hands; (2) Scanning the inner aura; (3) Sweeping or cleansing, general and localised; (4) Increasing the receptivity of the patient; (5) Energising with prana through the hand chakras technique by: (a) drawing in prana and (b) projecting prana; (6) Stabilizing the projected prana and (7) Releasing the projected pranic healing energy.

All these have been tried and tested and most people are able to produce positive results in just a few sessions by properly following the instructions, according to Choa Kok Sui, provided you maintain an open mind and persevere.

Sensitising the Hands

1. Place your hands about 3 inches apart facing each other. Do not tense, just relax.
2. Concentrate on feeling the centres of your palms. Try to be aware of the centres of your palms for

about 5 to 10 minutes while you inhale and exhale slowly and rhythmically. Concentration is made easier if you press the centre of your palms with your thumbs before starting. Concentration on the centre of the palms activates the and chakras thereby sensitizing the hands that is enabling them to feel the pranic energy or matter about 80 to 90% of those following this procedure will be able to feel a tingling sensation, heat, pressure, or rhythmic pulsation, between the palms at the first try. It is important to feel the pressure or rhythmic pulsation.

3. Proceed immediately to scanning (described below) after sensitizing your hands;

4. Practise sensitizing your hands for about a month. As a rule your hands should be more or less permanently sensitised after a month of practice.

5. Do not be discouraged if your don't feel anything after your first try. Continue your practice. It is likely that you will be able to feel this subtle sensation by the fourth session. It is essential to keep an open mind and concentrate on the procedure.

Scanning

In scanning, it is helpful but not essential to first learn how to feel the size and shape of the outer and health auras before scanning the inner aura. This makes the hands more sensitive. In healing, we are primarily interested in scanning the inner aura through which the trouble spots can be located. When scanning with you hands always concentrate on the centres of your palms, thereby activating and further enhancing the activation of the hand chakras.

Procedure for Scanning the Outer Aura:

1. Stand about four metres away from your subject

with your palms facing your subject and your arms slightly outstretched.

2. Slowly walk towards the subject, simultaneously try to feel with your sensitised hands the subjects outer aura. Concentrate on the centres of your palms when scanning.
3. Stop when you feel heat, a tingling sensation or a slight pressure. You are now feeling the outer aura. Try feeling the size and shape of the outer aura its width from head to waist, waist to feet and front to back. Usually it feels like an inverted egg, wider at the top then at the bottom.
4. It is essential that you gradually become aware of the aura in terms of its pressure so as to be more accurate in finding out the widths of the outer, health and inner auras.
5. The outer aura is usually about one meter in radius but sometimes it can be more than two metres wide. Some hyperactive children have outer auras as wide as three metres.

Scanning the Health Aura:

1. Having determined the size and shape of the outer aura move forward gradually still retaining the earlier position. Stop as soon as you feel the subtle sensation again. These may be slightly more intense sensations. It is the Health aura that you are sensing now.
2. Scan the subject from head to foot and front to back. Scan the right and the left sides. When the inner aura of the right and left sides of the body are scanned they should have about the same thickness. If one side is bigger or smaller than the other, then there is something wrong with it.
3. Special attention should be paid to the major chakras that is the vital organs and the spine.

Sometimes a portion of the spine is either congested or depleted even if the patient has no back complaints.

4. While scanning the throat area the chin should be raised to get a more accurate scanning, because the inner aura of the chin can interfere with the actual condition of the throat.
5. Scan the lungs from the back or the sides rather than the front to get accurate results.
6. Pay special attention to the solar plexus since many diseases of emotional origin affect the solar plexus chakra.

Interpretation of Inner Aura Scanning Results:

1. While you scan your patient you may notice hollows or protrusions in some areas of the patient's inner aura. Hollows are caused by pranic depletion. Usually because the surrounding meridians or chakra channels are partially or severely blocked, preventing fresh prana from elsewhere to flow freely and vitalise the depleted part. In pranic depletion the chakra in question is depleted and filled with dirty diseased bioplasmic matter and is also usually partially underactivated.
2. When the area protrudes, it means there is pranic or bioplasmic congestion. Excess prana and bioplasmic matter, in the area in question cause the surrounding meridians to be blocked so that the excess prana and bioplasmic matter cannot flow out freely. The affected chakra filled with diseased bioplasmic matter is usually over activated.
3. Some organ of the body may be affected by both pranic congestion and depletion simultaneously. This means that a portion of the affected organ is hollow while another is protruding.
4. The smaller the inner aura the more severe is the

pranic depletion. The bigger the protrusion of the aura the greater is the congestion of the affected part.

5. A part of the body may have a temporary pranic surplus in which case there is nothing wrong with the area as, for example, a person who has been sitting down for a long time when scanned may show a big protruson of the inner aura around the buttock area. But the condition normalises soon.

6. Similarly, a part of the body may experience temporary pranic reduction with nothing wrong in it. For example, a recent quarrel could have caused a temporary pranic reduction around the solar plexus area, which a few hours rest will normalise. But continuous or habitual anger may cause chronic pranic depletion around the solar plexus resulting in abdominal ailments and even heart disease.

7. The physical condition of the patient should be observed carefully and the patient questioned exhaustively before jumping to any conclusion.

8. Diseases manifest themselves first on the bioplasmic body before being experienced by the physical body. Therefore, pranic healing should be applied to the disease before it could be manifested physically.

Sweeping

Sweeping is used as a cleansing technique but can also be used for energising and distributing excess prana. Cleansing done for the whole bioplasmic body is termed general sweeping and when done on specific parts of the body is called localised sweeping. Both hands are used in sweeping, sometimes held in cup hand position and other times in spread-finger position. These positions are used alternately. The cupped hand position is effective for removing the deceased bioplasmic matter while the spread finger position is appropriate for combing and disentangling the health rays.

Localised Sweeping: This is done by: 1) Placing your one or both hands above the affected area. Concentrate on your hand and on the affected organ. Then slowly sweep away the deceased bioplasmic matter as if cleaning a dirty object with your hand; 2) Strongly flicking your hand to throw away the dirty bioplasmic matter; 3) The sweeping movements can be carried out vertically, horizontally diagonally or in an 'L' shaped movement; 4) For simple ailments localised sweeping should be done twenty to thirty times over the affected organ. Often the patient will feel partial or complete relief. This is a useful practice in treating stomach pain, loose bowel movement and headaches; 5) In case of more severe ailments the number of localised sweeping treatments should be increased. In case of cyst localised sweeping carried out fifty times is appropriate; in case of acute hepatitis about hundred or more sweepings may be necessary; in case of tumour or cancer it will have to be performed 300 to 500 times; and 6) Experienced and proficient pranic healers are able to get effective results with greatly reduced number of sweeping movements.

Sweeping is very easily learnt by most people. They should however take care that in localised sweeping the diseased bioplasmic matter is not transferred from one part of the body to another. In such a situation localised sweeping needs to be applied on the newly affected area.

General Sweeping: This is done with a series of downward sweeping movements only. Here you start from the head down to the feet. Upwards sweeping movements are not used in cleansing but to reawaken patients who may have fallen asleep or may have grown drowsy. In this case you start from the feet and go up to the head.

The General Sweeping Procedure is as Follows:

1. Cup your hands and place them six inches above the head of the patient. Don't touch the patient. Maintain a minimum distance of about two inches between your patient's body and your hands;
2. With your hands still cupped sweep your hands slowly downward. From head to foot. Slowly raise your hands and strongly flick them downwards to throw away the dirty diseased bioplasmic matter. This avoids recontaminating the patient with the diseased matter as also contaminating yourself;
3. Repeat the procedure (2) with spread-finger position instead of the cupped hand position. This disentangles and strenghtens the health rays and is called combing;
4. Repeat the whole process as in no. (2) and (3) to the sides of the patient.
5. Repeat the downward sweeping on the back of the patient. Using the same procedure as in nos. 2, 3 and 4;
6. It is essential to concentrate on the intention to remove the diseased bioplasmic matter. Otherwise the sweeping becomes less effective and more time consuming. With practice you can effectively use the sweeping movement with great ease and minimum effort.
7. Focus intention on the centres of your palms until the patient is sufficiently energised. In simple cases this may take about 5 -15 minutes for beginners.

There should be an initial intention to draw in prana through one hand chakra and to project it to the other. Once the initial intention has been established, there is no need to consciously maintain this intention. The position of the hands, initial intention and the concentration on the centre of the palms will cause prana to be drawn in automatically through one of the hand chakras and projected through the other.

Some healers commit the mistake of concentrating too much on the projecting hand and not enough on the receiving hand, and are not able to project enough pranic energy because they are not drawing enough of it. They also tend to become easily exhausted because they are using their own pranic energy instead of drawing it from the surroundings. Consequently, you should concentrate more on the receiving hand than on the projecting hand to avoid becoming depleted.

When energising or projecting prana you should form an initial intention of directing the projected prana to the affected chakra and only then to the affected part. It is critically important that the projected prana be directed at the affected part since it will produce a much faster rate of relief and healing. Just energising the affected chakra without directing the pranic energy to the affected part will result in a slower distribution of prana from the treated chakra to the affected part, producing a slower rate of relief and healing.

The right and left armpits should be slightly open to permit an easier flow of prana from one hand chakra to the other.

If you feel a slight pain or discomfort in your hand while energising, flick your hand to throw away the absorbed diseased bioplasmic matter. When energising the hand should be regularly flicked;

Energising should be continued till the treated part is sufficiently energised and you feel a slight repulsion from the treated part or a gradual cessation of flow of prana from your hand to the treated part. The flow of prana may feel like a warm or subtle moving current. For beginners energising 5-15 minutes for simple cases and about 30 minutes or more for more severe cases.

Cross check whether the treated area is sufficiently

energised by simply rescanning the inner aura of the treated part. If it is not then energise further until the treated part has sufficient prana.

If the treated part is over energised apply distributive sweeping to prevent possible pranic congention;

Prana can also be projected through the fingers or finger chakras rather than hand chakras. The prana coming out of the finger chakras is more intense and the patient may feel pain and a boring or penetrating sensation that is quite unnecessary. It is better to master energising through the hand chakras before trying to energise through the finger chakras.

One of the potential problems in pranic healing is the instability of the projected prana which tends to leak out gradually causing a recurrence of the illness. This can be prevented by stabilising the projected prana in two ways:

1. Complete all energising with prana by projecting blue prana. This is done by visualising and projecting light blue prana on the treated part;
2. Mentally instructing the projected prana to stabilize itself.

Now that you know to heal using pranic healing the following schedule should be maintained daily to acquire the necessary practice:

1. Sensitizing the hands—5 to 10 minutes a day;
2. Scanning—5 to 10 minutes a day;
3. General and localised sweeping—10 minutes a day; and
4. Energising with prana—10 minutes a day.

This schedule should be maintained for at least 5-10 weeks to prepare yourself to heal somebody like your own child or others of simple ailments like fever, lose bowel movement, gas pain, muscle pain, insect and bug bites... This technique should preferably be applied on actual patients but if they are not available practice with a friend or relative.

It is advisable to learn to heal simple ailments at least thirty times before proceeding to treat more difficult cases. It is also advisable to study Choa Kok Sui's *The Ancient Science and Art of Pranic Healing*. Although the basics have been given in the chapter to enable you to start on your own reading this book and his subsequent books particularly *Advanced Pranic Healing* will give you much greater confidence. Both these books contain specific treatments for specific ailments besides the general treatment which has been given here in a condensed fashion.

Index

J

Jain 3
—Doctors Association 1
—Doctors Federation 3-6
—Monks 4
Jainism 9
Jasmuheen 22, 24, 33, 53-54, 57-58,
 60-65, 67-68, 122
Jaundice 49
Jeff 63
Jesus 30, 141
Jian 41
Jitubhai Shah, Dr. 3
Joan Wester Anderson 59
Johann Steiner 32
Jungian psychology 58

K

Kabalah 56
Kachhi Jain Samaj 5
Karma 5
—pratyahara 171-172
Kelp 120-121
Kervan 122
Ketones 10
Key Genes 103
Ki 19, 133, 175
Kicharee 169
Kidney cleanse 119
—Failure 70
K.K. Shah, Dr. 5
Koshas 161
Kulviskas 125
Kundalini energy 154
—shakti 160
Kung 133
Kutchi 1

L

'L' shaped movement 180
Lack of protein 93
Lani Morris 77
LARGER medicine 123

Laser 50
Laurie Schoonhoven 37
Laxmiben Khona, Dr. 3
Laya Yoga 170
Layers Of Detoxification 141
Leonardo Da Vinci 148
Levitation 60
Life 31
—Energy 80, 133
—Force 71, 79, 124 , 132, 160
Light 49, 86
—Ambassadors 99, 101, 103, 104
—Body 154
—Eater 129
—of God 62
Linn 53
Lipid profiles 5
Liquids 120
—Light 34, 53, 57, 61
Liquidarian-s 34, 142
Living on Light 19, 34, 36, 45, 53, 61,
 75, 105, 109, 110, 111, 112
Loath 77
Localised sweeping 180
Longevity 79
Loose bowel movement 180
Lotus position 55
Low Level Light Therapy (LLLT) 50
Lu Zuyin 94
Lungs 48
Luster 17

M

Mad Cow Disease 122
Madonna 56
Magnesiums 123
Magnetic Field-s 81-82
—Intensity 81
Malnutrition 18
Mano-pratyahara 172-173
Manobhakshi Aahar 15
Mantra 173
Massachusetts Institute of Technol-
 ogy 38

SOME MORE NAB PUBLICATIONS

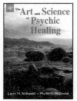
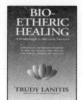

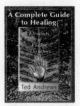

A COMPLETE GUIDE TO HEALING — *Ted Andrews*
With the help of this book you can take your first steps toward developing your innate ability to heal. The straightforward techniques detailed here will serve to pinpoint what you can control in yourself, what you need to learn about yourself, and what you need to change to become healthier on all levels: emotional, mental, spiritual and physical.

ISBN: 81-7822-119-5

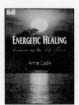

ENERGETIC HEALING — *Arnie Lade*
Energetic Healing is a guide to the inner landscape of subtle energy. In this ground-breaking book the role, manifestation, utility and healing power of our life force/energy is explored in a concise and informative fashion. Furthermore, a compelling and original model of energy is provided, one that bridges many seemingly separate disciplines to reveal their unity and usefulness. Discover for yourself the unique expression of energy that binds body, mind and spirit together.

ISBN: 81-7822-005-9

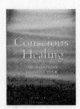

CONSCIOUS HEALING — *John Selby*
Based on new medical research and on their extraodinary success in teaching sick people how to activate and balance their own immune systems, therapist John Selby and Manfred von Lühmann MD, offer twelve mind-body methods that provide anyone suffering from an illness or injury with step-by-step programme for inner self-healing to supplement a doctor's care. It also includes invaluable information for maintaining health and wellness by boosting your immune system through conscious healing.

ISBN: 81-7822-157-8

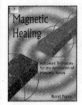

MAGNETIC HEALING — *Buryl Payne*
Through this book you can discover the positive benefits of magnetism for improving your health and well-being. The book narrates: what ailments can be treated with magnets; how do magnets work to heal the body; which polarity should be used for which condition; what is the correct way to use magnets; how long should magnets be placed on the body; what are the latest magnetic health products now being used; etc.

ISBN: 81-7822-002-4

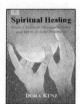

SPIRITUAL HEALING — *Dora Kunz*
Healing is a divine art. The book presents a surprising open-mindedness and forward looking vision. A spiritual revolution is underway in health care. More and more doctors, nurses, and counselors are recognizing that health means treating the soul and the psyche as well as the body. In this new edition of a classic collection, the best minds in holistic healing explore the spiritual basis of the alternative health care movement.

ISBN: 81-7822-011-3

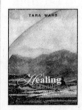

THE HEALING HANDBOOK—*Tara Ward*
This will help you to revitalise your life force. Many people view healing as a purely physical experience while many others rely dealing with the whole person and acknowledging the connection between the physical, mental, emotional and spiritual aspects of the self. Spiritual healing can be very effective on a basic level and presents a range of techniques and tools for healing yourself and others, including children and animals.

ISBN: 81-7822-034-2